Recent Advances in Pancreatitis

Edited by Qiang Yan

Published in London, United Kingdom

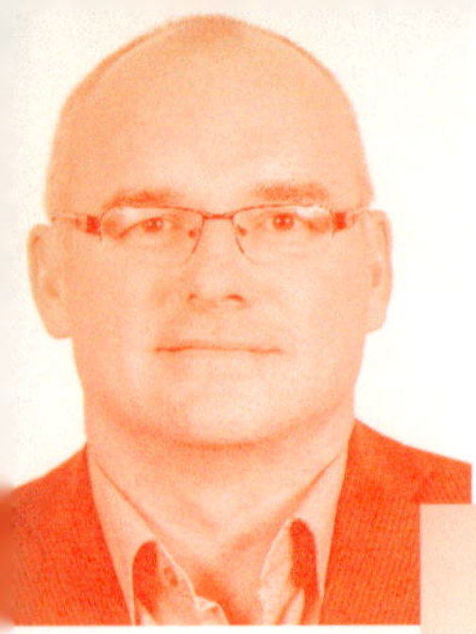
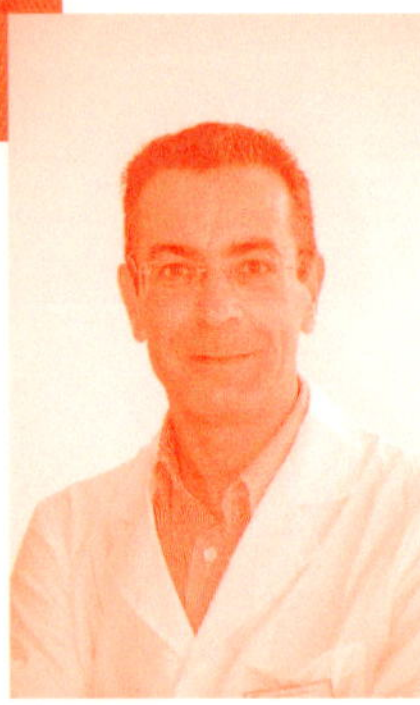
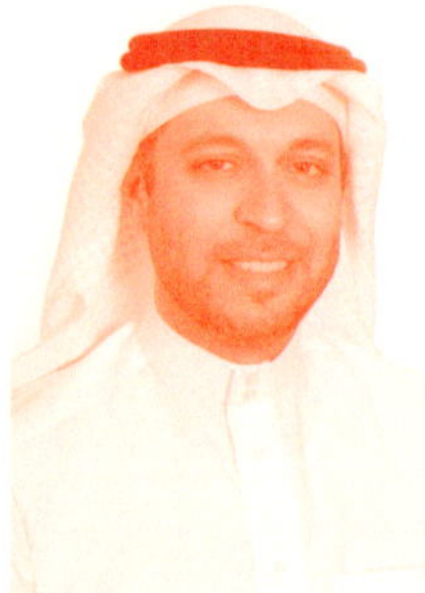
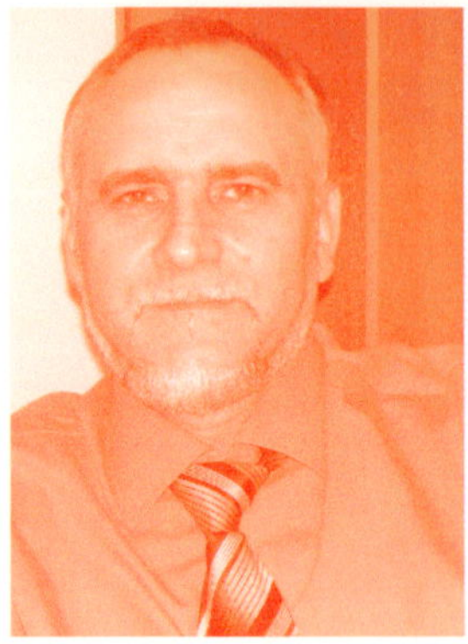
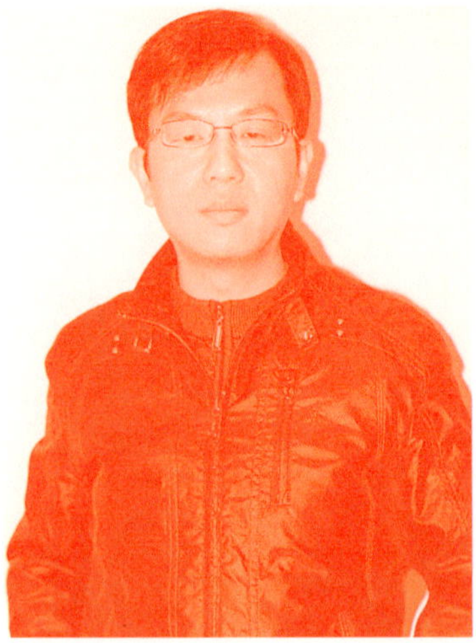
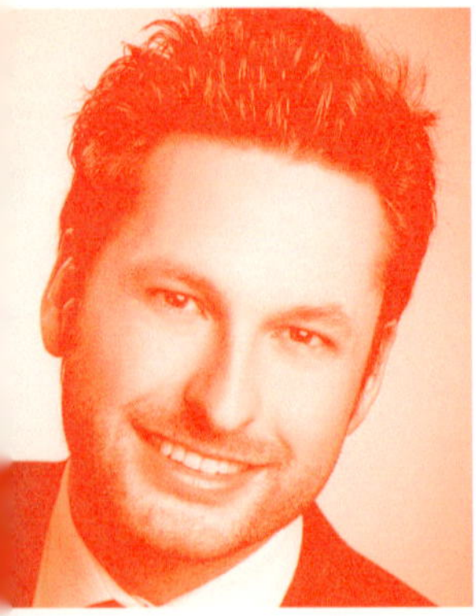
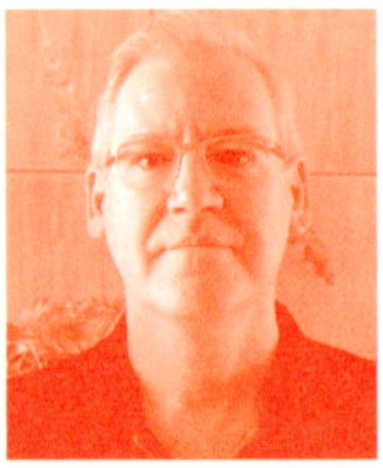

IntechOpen

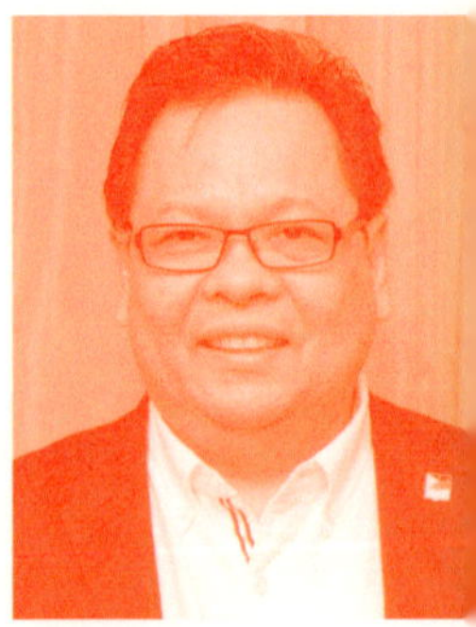
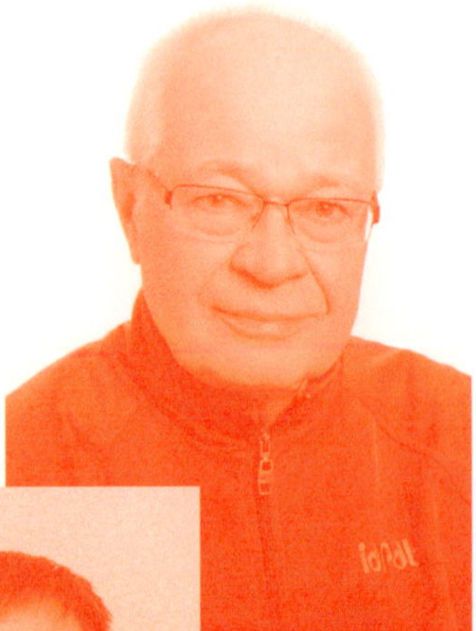
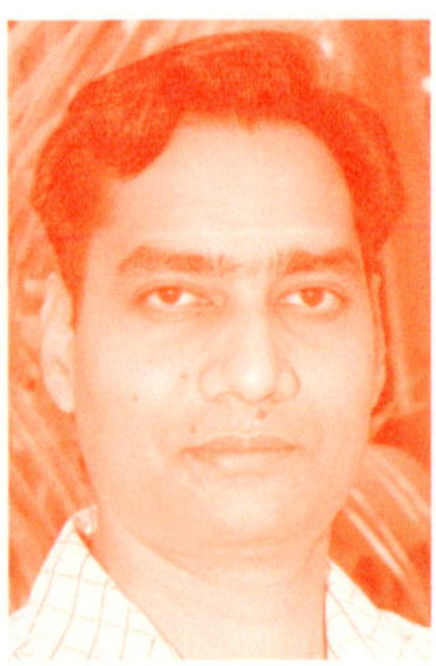
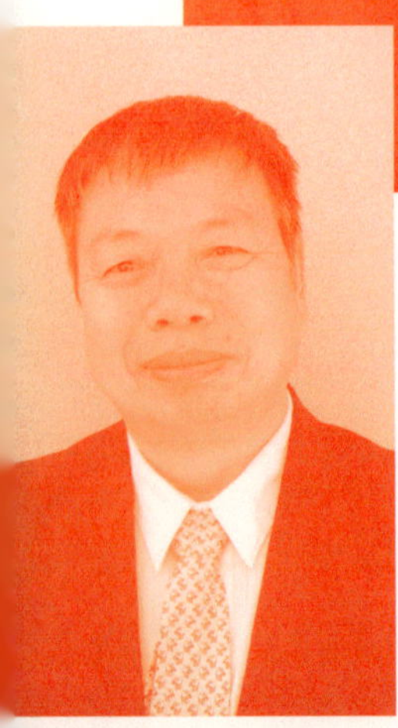
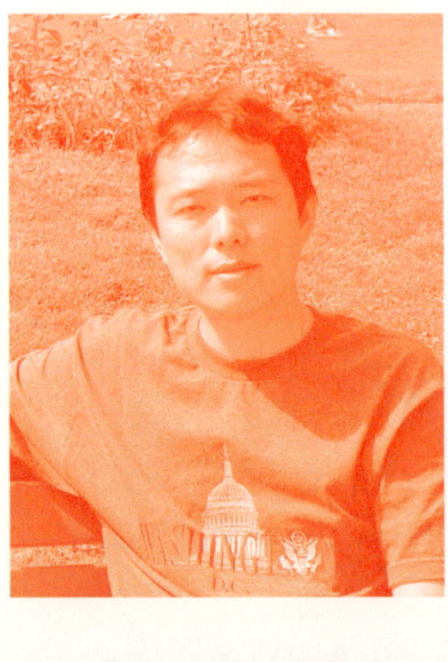
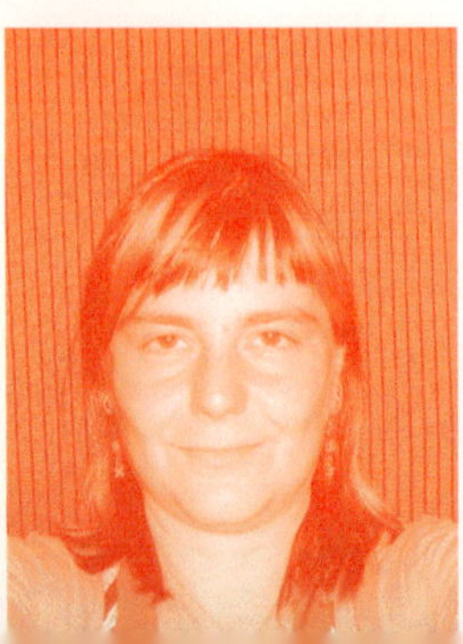

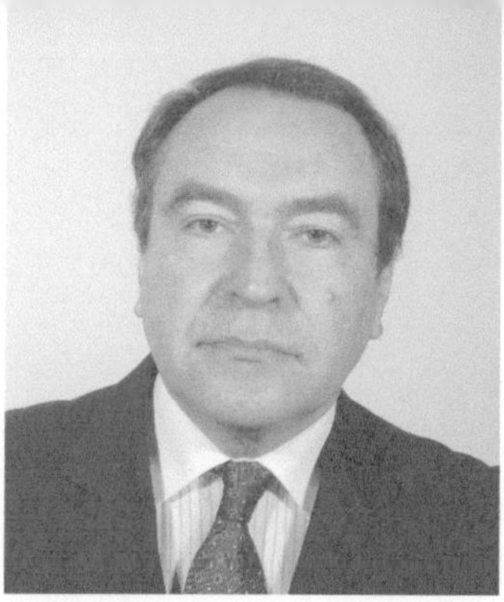
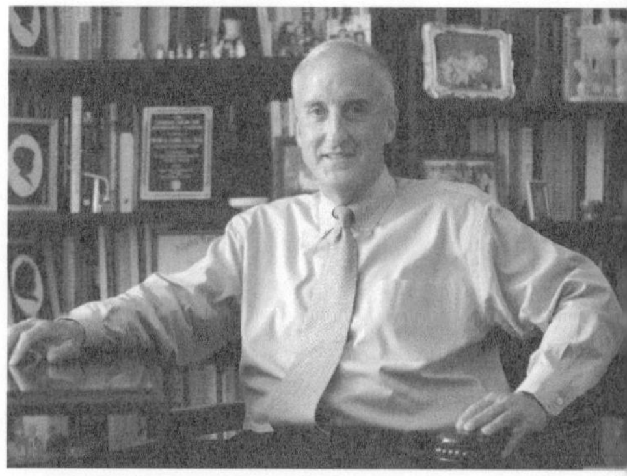
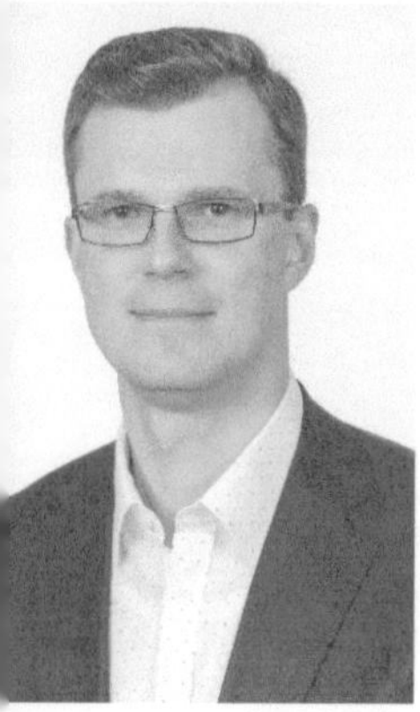
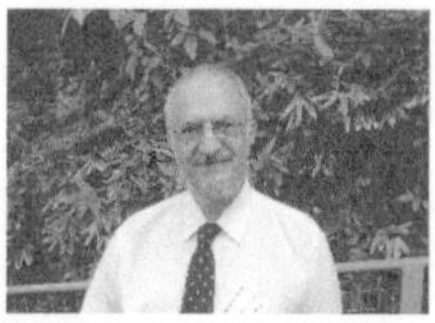
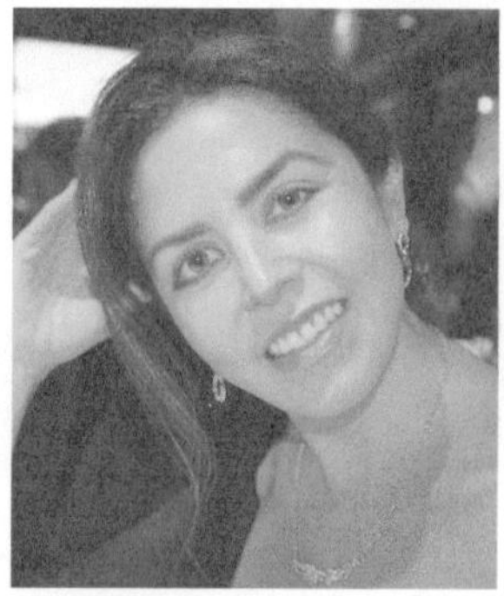

Supporting open minds since 2005

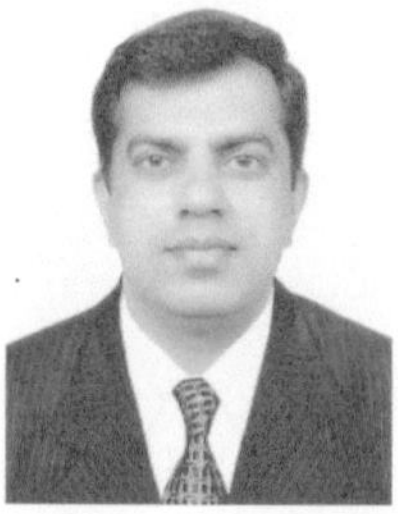
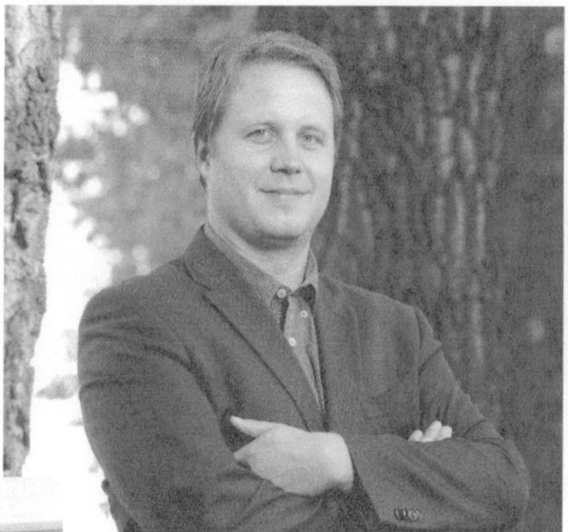
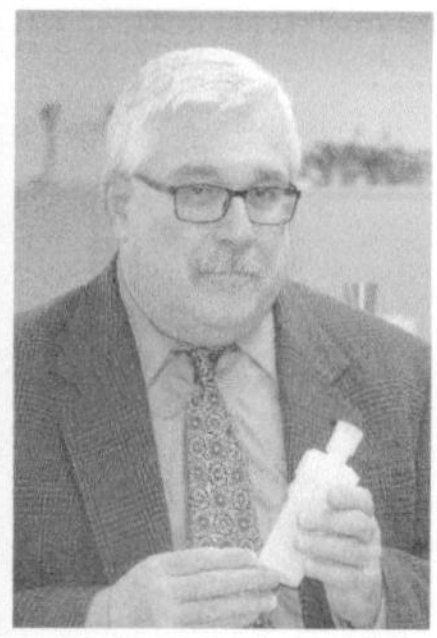
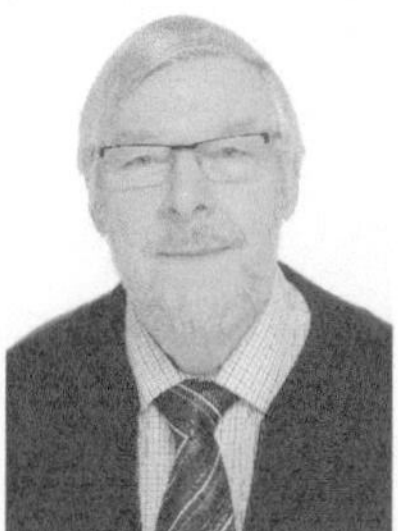
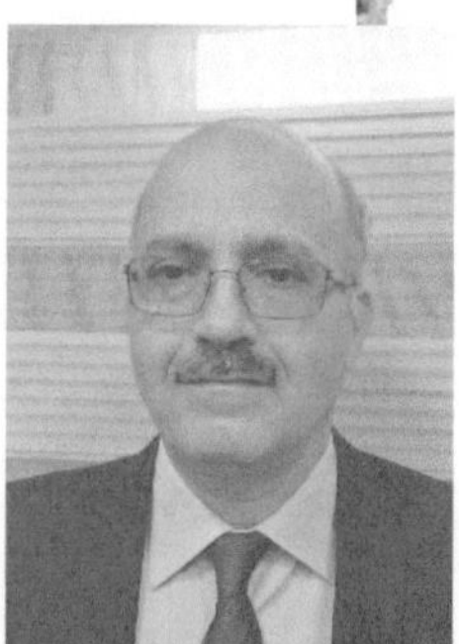
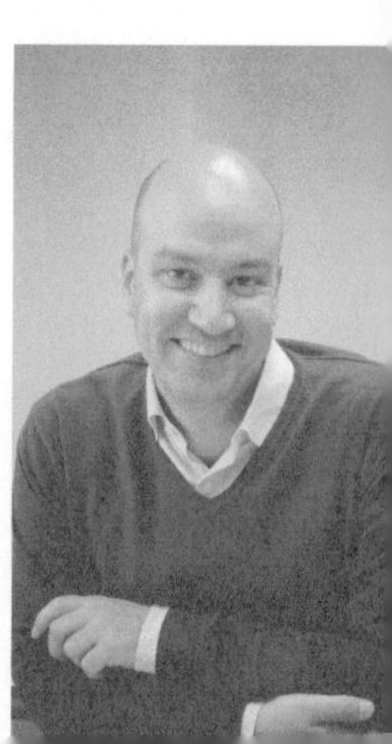
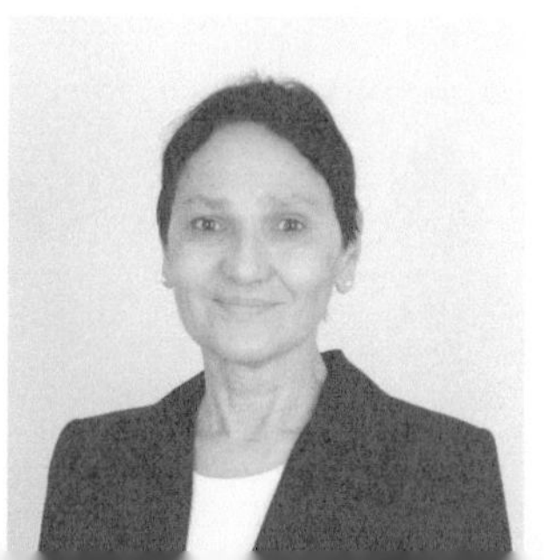

Recent Advances in Pancreatitis
http://dx.doi.org/10.5772/intechopen.91504
Edited by Qiang Yan

Assistant to the Editor: Zhenhua Shen

Contributors
Betsabé Reyes, Javier Padilla, Pilar Elena González, Pablo Sanz, Matthew Giangola, Dane Thompson, Siavash Bolourani, Rezan Karaali, Firdevs Topal, Tommaso Stecca, Bruno Pauletti, Luca Bonariol, Ezio Caratozzolo, Enrico Battistella, Silvia Zilio, Marco Massani, Didem Saka, Gürhan Şişman, Elif Reyyan Çadırcıbaşı, Can Boynukara, Ülkü Saritaş, Yücel Üstündağ

First published in London, United Kingdom, 2022 by IntechOpen
IntechOpen is the global imprint of INTECHOPEN LIMITED, registered in England and Wales, registration number: 11086078, 5 Princes Gate Court, London, SW7 2QJ, United Kingdom
Printed in Croatia

British Library Cataloguing-in-Publication Data
A catalogue record for this book is available from the British Library

Additional hard and PDF copies can be obtained from orders@intechopen.com

Recent Advances in Pancreatitis
Edited by Qiang Yan
p. cm.
Print ISBN 978-1-83968-898-0
Online ISBN 978-1-83968-899-7
eBook (PDF) ISBN 978-1-83968-900-0

For EU product safety concerns:
IN TECH d.o.o., Prolaz Marije Krucifikse Kozulić 3, 51000 Rijeka, Croatia, info@intechopen.com or visit our website at intechopen.com.

Meet the editor

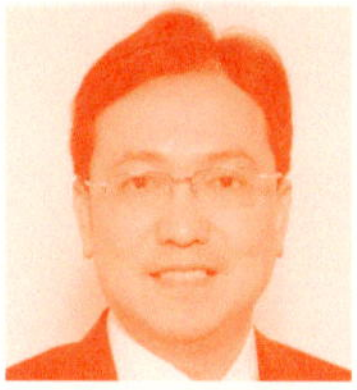

Qiang Yan, MD, Ph.D., FACS, is a Professor of Surgery and Vice President of Affiliated Huzhou Hospital, Zhejiang University School of Medicine (Huzhou Central Hospital). He is a senior hepato-pancreatic-biliary (HPB) surgeon. Dr. Yan is the academic leader of the Department of General Surgery and Division of Hepatopancreatic and Biliary Surgery, Huzhou Central Hospital (North Zhejiang Provincial General Surgery Center) and the academic leader of Huzhou municipal clinical research center of the malignant tumor. He is also executive vice president of the Huzhou Anticancer Association. Dr. Yan joined the Department of Surgery in 1997. He became the director of the Division of HPB Surgery in 2009 and chairman of the Department of Surgery in 2015. He undertook special training at the Department of HPB and Minimally Invasive Surgery, Universität of Regensburg, Germany, in 2009 and Stanford University, USA in 2012. He received his Surgical Leadership Program certification from Harvard Medical School, USA, in 2019. Professor Yan became a fellow of the American College of Surgery in 2016 and a special member of the Japan–Germany Society of Study of Liver Surgery in 2018. He is now an active member of the *HPB* journal, the Gastrointestinal Physicians branch of World Endoscopy Doctors Association, Chinese College of Surgeons, Chinese Medical Doctor Association, Zhejiang Medical Doctor Association, Surgery, Chinese Medical Association Zhejiang Branch. He is also deputy director of the Zhejiang Invention Association Endoscopic Branch and deputy president of the College of Surgeons. He is an executive guest editor of *Anti-Cancer Agents in Medicinal Chemistry* and an invited reviewer of medicine at Johns Hopkins Hospital and *Frontiers in Oncology*.

Contents

Preface

Pancreatitis is a common disease of the digestive system and one of the most common causes of death. Until relatively recently, pancreatitis has been extremely difficult to study and treat, and many problems of pancreatitis have not been clarified. The correct diagnosis of chronic pancreatitis at an early stage is difficult, and end-stage chronic pancreatitis or acute pancreatitis with extensive necrosis of the gland is tricky to treat. Within the past decade, revolutionary techniques in molecular biology and minimally invasive treatment have begun to give us dramatic new clinical tools for diagnosing and treating pancreatic disease. This book provides a comprehensive discussion of the anatomy and physiology of the pancreas, acute and chronic pancreatitis, and minimally invasive treatment in pancreatitis. It is hoped that this book will provide evidence for clinicians to make clinical decisions and provide scientists with a comprehensive overview of the current developments in this critically important area.

Qiang Yan
Department of General Surgery,
Huzhou Central Hospital,
Affiliated Huzhou Hospital,
Zhejiang University School of Medicine,
Huzhou, Zhejiang, China

Section 1

Acute and Chronic Pancreatitis

Chapter 1

Emergency Management of Acute Pancreatitis

Rezan Karaali and Firdes Topal

Abstract

Acute pancreatitis (AP) is the sudden inflammation of the pancreas, and it may be confined to the pancreas, or more life-threatening, affecting all organs and systems. AP is a common gastrointestinal condition Worldwide and is associated with cost to the health care system. It progresses mildly in 80% of patients and resolves with treatment, but in cases of severe AP, with mortality of around 30% recorded. In this section, we will discuss the first management of the AP in the emergency department. Because this is the period when management decisions can change the course of the disease and the length of stay in the hospital. In the management AP, approaches regarding the utility and timing of antibiotics, the timing and type of nutritional support, endoscopic retrograde cholangiopancreatography (ERCP) and cholecystectomy approaches are constantly being updated. Treatment is mainly related to the severity of the disease. With early diagnosis and treatment, most of the patients can be discharged, and the development of complications and mortality can be reduced. Therefore, emergency management is important in acute pancreatitis.

Keywords: acute pancreatitis, complications, diagnosis, emergency, management

1. Introduction

1.1 Definition and incidence

Acute pancreatitis (AP) refers to the sudden inflammation of the pancreas, and it may be confined to the pancreas, or more life-threatening, affecting all organs and systems [1–5]. Recurrence is experienced in 15–30% of patients, and 5–25% can develop chronic pancreatitis. It progresses mildly in 80% of patients and resolves with treatment, but in cases of severe AP, complications such as organ failure and pancreatic necrosis may develop, with mortality of around 30% recorded in this group [2, 4, 5]. AP is an acute gastrointestinal disease that requires hospitalization, and is the most common cause of admission to the emergency room worldwide [1, 6, 7]. Hospital admissions for AP in the United States are in the region of 270,000/year, with a mortality rate of 30% in severe cases. Death is due to systemic inflammatory response syndrome (SIRS) and organ failure in the first two weeks, while death after two weeks can be attributed to sepsis and complications [3, 6, 8, 9].

1.2 Etiology

Gallstones are the most common etiology of AP, being responsible for 40–70% of AP cases [10–12]. The ease at which small gallstones can pass into the bile duct make

AP more common in this patient group [13]. Although alcohol is commonly blamed as the second most common cause, the link between alcohol and AP is unclear, as AP is seen in only a small number of alcoholics [2, 14, 15]. Recent studies have suggested that alcohol increases the oxidative metabolism in the acinar cells of the pancreas, thereby causing mitochondrial dysfunction and cell death. This increases also the production of acetaldehyde in the pancreatic stellate cells, and increases circulating lipopolysaccharide and tumor necrosis factor alpha (TNFα), leading to fibrosis in the pancreas [16, 17]. Alcohol has also been reported to increase the viscosity of pancreatic juice and to cause ductal obstructions. That said, it has also been suggested that genetic factors play a role in the development of AP,based on the low incidence of AP in people with chronic alcohol consumption [2, 15, 18]. Other causes have been identified as Hypertriglyceridemia (HTR), and diabetes, hypothyroidism, pregnancy and obesity that cause HTR [1]. Patients with a body mass index (BMI) >35 are at risk of both HTR and AP, while those with serum triglyceride levels >1000 mg/dl are at greater risk [19–21]. Following endoscopic retrograde cholangiopancreatography (ERCP) performed by inexperienced practitioners, patients with Sphincter of Oddi dysfunctions may develop AP following ERCP due to difficult cannulation [22].

AP can also occur due to drugs at a rate of 0.1–0.5% [2, 23–25]. Many drugs have been identified that cause acute pancreatitis. Drugs cause AP by different mechanisms. While some drugs cause direct toxicity to the pancreas (eg, diuretics, sulfonamides), some drugs cause acute pancreatitis by causing an immunological reaction (eg, 6-mercaptopurine, amino salicylates, sulfonamides). Diuretics and azothiopurine cause direct ischemia, while hormones such as steroids and estrogen cause vascular thrombosis or ischemic pancreatitis by decreasing the viskosity of the pancreatic juice. Toxic metabolites of drugs such as valproic acid and tetracycline may accumulate in the pancreas and cause pancreatitis [2, 26, 27].

AP cases have been reported associated with such infectious diseases as Mumps, Coxsackievirus, Hepatitis B, Cytomegalovirus, Varicella-Zoster, herpes simplex and human immunodeficiency virus (HIV) among the viruses; with Mycoplasma, Legionella, Leptospira and Salmonella among the bacteria; with Aspergillus among the fungi; and with Toxoplasma and Cryptosporidium among the parasites [2, 27, 28]. There have been reports of cases of AP with the recent SARS-CoV-2 infection at the heart of the current global pandemic [29, 30]. In a review of current literature, AP was found to be detected in 17% of patients hospitalized due to Covid-19 [29]. Although tests for specific infectious agents are not generally recommended in AP patients, Covid-19 infection should also be kept in mind in AP cases during the pandemic [30].

Concerning other rare causes, pancreatic injury following trauma is an extremely rare condition due to its retroperitoneal nature. Pancreatic duct injuries may occur due to blunt or penetrating traumas [31], while AP may occur due to gallbladder sludge, tumors, autoimmune pancreatitis, hypercalcemia, anatomical and physiological anomalies (pancreatic divisum, biliary cysts, pancreaticobiliary malunion, large juxta-ampullary diverticula, annular pancreas and Sphincter of Oddi dysfunction), and vasculitis [27, 32–36]. Ischemic AP can also be seen after major cardiovascular operations [27, 37, 38]. Patients with an unknown etiology after history-taking, physical examination, laboratory tests, imaging methods and advanced tests are classified as idiopathic. In the event of recurrent AP attacks in this patient group and AP at a young age, genetic factors should be investigated [27, 39].

1.3 Pathogenesis

As its main mechanism, AP blockades the secretion of enzymes while the synthesis of enzymes continues [2, 40]. Under normal conditions, trypsinogen is produced in the pancreas and secreted into the duodenum where it is converted into protease trypsin, but in cases where secretion is blocked, trypsin continues to be produced in pancreatic acinar cells. While activation continues, elimination is inhibited, and the active trypsin damages the vascular endothelium, interstitium and acinar cells [2, 40, 41]. As a result, autodigestion begins in the pancreas,and ischemia occurs at a tissue level in the pancreas due to the vasoconstriction and stasis of the capillary vessels. The activation of granulocytes and macrophages in response to these events causes a release of proinflammatory cytokines (tumor necrosis factor, interleukins 1, 6 and 8), arachidonic acid metabolites (prostaglandins, platelet activating factor and leukotrienes), proteolytic and lipolytic enzymes, and reactive oxygen metabolites [2, 27, 42, 43]. All of these factors together cause damage to the pancreatic tissue. In general, the inflammation is locally self-limiting, buton occasions, inflammatory agents may cause a systemic response, leading to the damage and failure of distant organs. This, in turn, may result in Acute Respiratory Distress Syndrome (ARDS), pleural effusion, acute renal failure, shock, and even death [2, 27, 44, 45].

2. Clinical features

Patients withAP present to the emergency room with sudden and severe abdominal pain that usually starts in the epigastric region. In patients with gallstones, the pain spreads to the right upper quadrant and is more sharply limited. In 50% of patients, the pain spreads to the back, and is felt around the entire abdomen, like a belt. Nausea and vomiting may accompany,and in rare cases there may be pain on the left side of the abdomen [2, 46–49].

Physical examination findings can vary, depending on the severity of AP and any accompanying diseases. Initial findings typically include mild or generalized tenderness upon abdominal palpation, distension and diminished bowel sounds. In cases of obstruction due to gallstones, jaundice may be observed, while in severe AP, fever, hypotension, tachycardia, tachypnea and hypoxemia may be observed. In cases of pancreatic necrosis, ecchymotic lesions can be seen in the periumbilical region (Cullen's sign) or on the flanks (Gray Turner's sign) [2, 27, 50, 51].

3. Diagnosis

Diagnosis is established based on the presence of two of three criteria: 1) Presence of clinical findings consistent with AP, 2) serum lipase or amylase levels three times greater than normal, and 3) characteristic findings of AP on imaging [2, 27, 47, 48, 52].

3.1 Laboratory

In AP, enzymes pass from the basolateral membrane to the interstitial area, and then on to the systemic circulation due to the blockade of the secretion ofpancreatic enzymes, while the synthesis of enzymes continues, resulting in increased levels of pancreatic enzymes in the blood.

At the onset of AP, serum amylase starts to increase within 6–12 hours, peaks at 48 hours, and returns to normal within 3–5 days, although no increase in amylase levels will be observed in alcohol-induced pancreatitis and AP due to hypertriglyceridemia. Sensitivity and specificity in diagnosis are 67–83% and 85–98%, respectively [2, 27, 48, 53, 54]. Elevated amylase levels may also be seen in non-pancreatic diseases, such as renal failure, salivary gland diseases, acute appendicitis, cholecystitis, perforations, intestinal obstructions or intestinal ischemia, and gynecological diseases. For these reasons, amylase alone is not sufficient for a diagnosis of AP [2, 48, 49]. The increase in serum lipase levels in AP is more specific. Following the onset of symptoms, the levels begin to increase within 8–10 hours, peak at 24 hours, return to normal within 8–14 days, with a sensitivity of 82–100% [2, 48, 53, 55], and may increase in alcohol-induced AP and AP due to hypertriglyceridemia. It is useful in delayed patients who present 24 hours after the onset of pain [48, 55, 56]. Aside from amylase-lipase, liver and kidney tests,a complete blood count should also be made in AP, as this will allow the assessment of the patient's clinical condition, the early identification of complications and the detection of organ failure, and will aid in a therapeutic evaluation. An alanine aminotransferase (ALT) liver function test value in excess of 150 U/L indicates gallstones [2, 47, 52]. There are also specific tests for AP that are not routinely used. Among the enzymes with early elevation are trypsinogen-activating peptide, urinary and serum trypsinogen and trypsin, phospholipase, carboxypeptidase, carboxyl ester lipase, colipase and pancreatic isoamylase [57–59], and an increase is also observed in inflammatory mediators such as C-reactive protein (CRP), interleukin IL-6, IL-8, IL-10, tumor necrosis factor (TNF) and PMN elastase. The elevation of inflammatory mediators is usually proportional to the severity of AP. A CRP level above 150 mg/dl within the first 48 hours has been associated with severe AP [60, 61].

3.2 Imaging

Imaging can aid in determining the etiology of AP, or complications due to AP. Abdominal and chest radiographs may reveal appearances of pleural effusion, atelectasis and ileus accompanying AP. Radiographs should be evaluated to rule out other causes of abdominal pain. Abdominal ultrasound should be performed on every patient with suspected AP, and USG can detect findings that support AP, if present, such as gallstones, obstructions in the common bile duct, intraabdominal free fluid and diffuse enlarged and hypoechoic appearance in the pancreas, as well as peripancreatic fluid, necrosis and abscesses. A normal USG cannot exclude AP [2, 27, 47, 48, 52, 62], while Contrast-Enhanced Computed Tomography (CECT) has a sensitivity of 90% in the diagnosis of AP. However, AP is not routinely recommended for diagnosis, since it is mild and uncomplicated in most patients [2, 47, 48, 52], but may be recommended in cases where other causes of acute abdomen cannot be excluded, or for patients who show no improvement within 48–72 hours [48, 63, 64].

Among the patients considered for CECT, MRI is recommended rather that CECT for those with renal failure, pregnant patients and those with allergies to IV contrast agents [48, 63].

Serum triglyceride levels must be examined in patients with normal test results, but with a strong suspicion of AP, in those with pancreatic tumors aged over 40 years, in the presence of genetic factors in patients under the age of 30 and in recurrent AP cases [39, 48].

3.3 Differential diagnosis

Other diseases that may cause abdominal pain should be excluded in a differential diagnosis.In particular, peptic ulcer disease, choledocholithiasis, cholangitis, biliary obstruction, cholecystitis, perforated viscus, intestinal obstruction, mesenteric ischemia and hepatitis should be considered in differential diagnosis due to their clinical similarities to AP [2, 27].

4. Initial management

AP can be classified into two groups as mild AP, in which patients have no accompanying organ failure, and recover and can be orally fed within 48 hours; and severe AP, which is accompanied by organ failure and a lack of response to treatment. Most patients with severe AP have not suffered organ failure at the time of admission to emergency room, and so may be evaluated as mild AP,but deteriorate rapidly due to inadequate hydration and inadequate treatment. As such, the severity of the disease should be determined along at the time of diagnosis in the emergency room, and treatment should be planned accordingly [47, 48, 52, 65].

According to the Atlanta classification, severe AP is characterized by resistant/persistent organ failure with no improvement within 48 hours, although in the absence of organ failure, the presence of local complications alone is an indicator of severe AP [66]. Patients who develop transient organ failure alongside local complications are classified as moderately severe AP (**Table 1**). The Atlanta classification evaluates the presence of organ failure based on Marshall's organ failure criteria. Accordingly, the presence of shock (systolic BP <90 mmHg), pulmonary failure (PaO2 < 60 mmHg), renal failure (creatinine >2 despite adequate hydration), and/or the presence of gastrointestinal bleeding (>500 ml blood loss within 24 hours) should be evaluated as organ failure [48, 52, 67].

Besides the Atlanta classification, several scoring systems have been proposed for the determination of the severity in AP. These include Ranson's criteria,Acute Physiology and Chronic Health Examination-II, modified Glasgow score, Bedside Index for Severity in Acute Pancreatitis and the Balthazar CT Severity Index,none of which has been shown to be superior to any other, and they have only limited use in the emergency room, as they rely on too many parameters, and some give results only after 48 hours [68, 69]. The assessment of the patient in the emergency department is of utmost importance, with patient-related risk factors such as age, weight, comorbidities and vital signs as well as laboratory findings all being evaluated together (**Table 2**) [47, 52, 56, 65].

Mild AP	Moderately AP	Severe AP
Absence of local complications	**Local complications** Peripancreatic fluid collection Pancreatic or peripancreatic necrosis(sterile or infected) Gastric outlet disfunction Splenic or portal vein thrombosis Colonic necrosis AND/OR	**Persistent organ failure > 48 h** GI bleeding (>500 cc/24 hr) Shock – SBP < 90 mmHg PaO 2 < 60% Creatinine >2 mg/d
Absence of organ failure	**Transient organ failure < 48 h**	
	GI bleeding (>500 cc/24 hr) Shock – SBP < 90 mmHg PaO 2 < 60% Creatinine >2 mg/d	

Table 1.
Atlanta classification 2015.

Patient characteristics	The systemic inflammatory response syndrome (SIRS)	Laboratory findings	Radiology findings
Age > 55 years Obesity (BMI >30 kg/m2) Altered mental status Comorbid disease	• pulse >90 beats/min • respirations >20/min or PaCO2 > 32 mmHg • temperature > 38°C or < 36°C • WBC count >12,000 or < 4,000 cells/mm3 or > 10% immature neutrophils (bands)	BUN >20 mg/dl Rising BUN HCT >44% Rising HCT Elevated creatinine	Pleural effusions Pulmonary infiltrates Multiple or extensive extrapancreatic collections

Table 2.
Initial assessment for risk of severe AP.

5. Treatment

5.1 Fluid replacement

The initial approach to AP involves aggressive fluid therapy, pain management and nutritional support. In AP, there is a large amount of fluid deficit due to losses from vomiting, reduced oral intake, passage of fluid into the third space, respiration and sweating. If the patient has no additional cardiovascular or renal disease, fluid replacement should be initiated at 5–10 ml/kg/hour. For patients presenting with evidence of hypovolemia and shock, 3 ml/kg of fluid should be given for 8–12 hours following a fluid bolus of 20 ml/kg in 30 minutes, with isotonic normal saline preferred as the fluid [47, 48, 52, 70–72]. A prospective study found hydration with Ringer's lactate solution to be more beneficial, although Ringer's lactate solution has been shown to activate trypsin in acinar cells, thereby making the patient more susceptible to injury due to its low pH. With normal saline, there is a risk of developing non-anion gap metabolic acidosis, and patients should be monitored accordingly during fluid replacement [2, 72]. An assessment should be made after 6, 24 and 48 hours to as certain whether the fluid administered is sufficient. With adequate hydration, the heart rate should drop below 120/min, mean arterial pressure (MAP) should be maintained between 65 and 85, and hematocrit (HCT) should be 35–44%. If the BUN value is initially high, a decrease upon hydration is an indicator of adequate hydration. Changes in blood urea nitrogen (BUN) values within the first 24 hours are particularly important [27, 47, 48, 73, 74]. If the BUN values continue to be high, or increase even further, acute tubular necrosis or resistant volume deficit should be suspected [27, 47, 52, 65, 75]. Another parameter that should be monitored during hydration is hematocrit. Continued hemoconcentration for more than 24 hours suggests the development of necrotizing pancreatitis, and so the patient's urine output, BUN and HCT values should be closely monitored. The development of severe pancreatitis should be considered in patients who do not respond to aggressive hydration for 6–12 hours [47, 48, 52].

5.2 Pain management

Adequate hydration and the resolution of hypovolemia relieve ischemic pain secondary to hemoconcentration. Nevertheless, opioid analgesics are recommended for rapid pain management. Fentanyl can be used safely, especially in patients with kidney failure, in which intravenous (IV) fentanyl of 20–50 microgram is administered slowly over 10 minutes. Meperidine can be used as an alternative to morphine due to the spasm effect of morphine on the Sphincter of Oddi [2, 27, 76, 77].

Vital signs	Laboratuary findings	Patient condition
pulse <40 or > 150 beats/min; systolic arterial pressure < 80 mmHg (<10.7 kPa) or mean arterial pressure < 60 or diastolic arterial pressure > 120 mmHg respiratory rate > 35 breaths/ min;	serum sodium <110 mmol/l or > 170 mmol/l; serum potassium<2.0 mmol/l or > 7.0 mmol/l; paO2 < 50 mmHg pH < 7.1 or > 7.7; serum glucose >800 mg/dl (>44.4 mmol/L); mmol/L); serum calcium >15 mg/dl (>3.75	coma. Furthermore, a patient with severe acute pancreatitis as defined by the revised Atlanta Classification (i.e. persistent organ failure)

Table 3.
Assessment for intensive care.

5.3 Monitoring

AP patients should be followed closely for 24 hours, with continued monitoring of blood pressure, temperature, pulse, oxygen saturation and urine output. Blood tests should be monitored for hematocrit, BUN and electrolytes (calcium, magnesium), and blood glucose should be maintained between 180 and 200 mg/dl [2, 27, 52]. Intensive care follow-up is required for patients whose vital signs and laboratory values are unstable and / or continue (**Table 3**) [52].

5.4 Nutrition

It is no longer recommended to stop oral intake until the AP has fully resolved and the enzymes have returned to normal limits in order to put the pancreas at rest. Patients ceasing oral intake may develop atrophy in the mucosa of gastrointestinal tract [27, 47, 48, 52, 78, 79], and so oral feeding should be initiated in patients without nausea, vomiting or ileus and with relieved pain, as soon as they can tolerate [47, 48, 52, 79–81]. Liquid, light and low-fat foods should be given at first [82]. In cases of severe AP, enteral feeding may be initiated in patients who are still unable to tolerate oral feeding after 5 days, and in those with complications. For enteral nutrition, a nasojejunal or nasogastric tube should be used for feeding. A nasogastric tube insertion may be easy, but there is a risk of aspiration, while a nasojejunal tube requires an operation. Depending on the conditions, both methods can help provide effective nutrition [47, 48, 82]. If the goal of enteral nutrition is not achieved within 48–72 hours, or if the patient cannot tolerate, parenteral nutrition should be initiated [80, 81, 83].

5.5 Antibiotics

20% of patients develop extrapancreatic infections that may be cholangitis, catheter infection, urinary tract infection or pneumonia. Prophylactic ABs, even if severe, are not routinely recommended in AP without an unidentified focus of infection or presence of infection. ABs for infective necrosis prophylaxis are not recommended, even for patients with sterile necrosis [2, 27, 47, 48, 52, 65, 84, 85].

6. Management of complications

If, during the follow-up of moderately severe or severe AP patients, signs of sepsis appear, no improvement occurs within 72 hours or the condition deteriorates gradually, then complications should be suspected and a CECT should be performed.

6.1 Local complications

6.1.1 Acute peripancreatic fluid collection

Acute peripancreatic fluid collection occurs early, and has no specific wall. It resorbs spontaneously [27, 48].

6.1.2 Necrotizing pancreatitis

Necrotizing pancreatitis can involve both the pancreas and peripancreatic tissues. A variable amount of fluid and necrotic tissue may develop within the necrosis,and is known as Acute Necrotic Collection (ANC) when a clear wall cannot be defined, and as Wall-off Necrosis (WON) when there is a mature, encapsulated and well-defined wall. WON is a pancreatic pseudocyst that occurs around 4 weeks after an AP attack, and that has a noticeable wall, for which drainage may be required. In either case, the necrotic area may be sterile or infected, and the type of treatment is determined based on the presence or absence of infection [84, 86–88].

6.1.2.1 Infected necrosis

Infection should be suspected in patients with pancreatic or extrapancreatic necrosis upon clinical deterioration or a lack of improvement within 7–10 days of hospitalization. Infectious agents are usually of intestinal origin (such as Escherichia coli, Pseudomonas, Klebsiella and Enterococcus), and may be suspected with the emergence of clinical signs of infection in patients and the presence of gas around the pancreas on imaging [89, 90]. Empirical AB may be initiated in these patients, with ABs that can penetrate the pancreas well (carbapenem alone; or quinolone, ceftazidime, or cefepime combined with an anaerobic agent such as metronidazole)being recommended [27, 47, 48]. Fine needle aspiration (FNA) or sampling is not recommended in such patients. Necrosectomy may be scheduled for patients who show no improvement, but should be delayed as much as possible, since many patients respond well to AB therapy [48, 90–92]. Antibiotic therapy should have been completed 4 weeks prior to a decision of necrosectomy. For the necrestomy, endoscopic or invasive percutaneous procedures should be tried first, and if these fail, surgery should be scheduled [47, 48, 52, 91–93].

6.1.2.2 Sterile necrosis

In patients with necrotizing pancreatitis, sterile necrotizing pancreatitis should be suspected when there is no improvement despite treatment, and no clear clinical or imaging findings of infection. In such cases, FNA sampling is indicated, and if the collected material is sterile, there is no need to continue the ABs. Even ABs cannot prevent sterile necrosis from turning into infected necrosis [47, 52, 94]. In sterile necrosis in the absence of any sign of infection, interventions will be required in the following cases:

- Continued obstruction of the gastric outlet, intestine or bile ducts, caused by mass effects after 4–8 weeks following the onset of acute pancreatitis.

- Persistant symptoms (e.g. abdominal pain, nausea, vomiting, anorexia or weight loss) identified more than eight weeks following the onset of acute pancreatitis.

- Disconnected duct syndrome (full transection of the pancreatic duct) with persistent symptomatic collections with necrosis (e.g., pain, obstruction) more than 8 weeks following the onset of acute pancreatitis.

Aside from these, CT and FNA should be repeated 5–7 days later in patients with sterile necrosis detected by CECT and FNA, but with signs of systemic toxicity [18, 52].

The much rarer complications include peripancreatic vascular complications, splanchnic vein thrombosis, abdominal compartment syndrome and pseudoaneurysm. Furthermore, patients may risk developing diabetes in the following periods [27, 52, 95].

6.2 Systemic complications

Respiratuar insufficiency includes pneumonia, atelectasis, and ARDS. Renal complications are prerenal azotemia, hypotansion and acute tubuler necrosis. Shock is caused by third space losses, vomiting and interstitial edema. Hypo-hyperglicemia, coagulation disorders, fat necrosis and pancreatic encphalophaty are other rare systemic complications of AP [27].

7. Management of predisposing underlying conditions

7.1 Nonsurgical management

The detection and treatment of the underlying diseases that cause AP are as important as AP itself. Most gallstones that pass into the common bile duct advance to the intestines, and are excreted with feces. However, stones that cause obstructions to the pancreatic duct and/or biliary ducts may result in severe AP and/or cholangitis. ERCP is recommended within the first 24 hours for AP patients with stones detected as causing an obstruction. The removal of stones by via a sphincterotomy with ERCP prevents both severe AP and the cholangitis and future development of biliary AP. ERCP should be performed within the first 24 hours in AP patients due to gallstones accompanied by acute cholangitis. A papillotomy, or the surgical removal of stones, with ERCP reduces the severity of AP [48, 52, 96–98]. It has been reported that mortality decreases with early ERCP in patients with no cholangitis, with biliary duct obstructions, and with elevated liver function test scores. That said, it is unnecessary to perform ERCP within the first 24 hours on patients with no increase in liver function tests, with therapeutic ERCP recommended for such patients before or during the cholecystectomy. It is recommended that EUS and MRCP be performed prior to ERCP in patients without cholangitis or jaundice, but with suspected choledocholithiasis, pregnant women and patients on whom ERCP cannot be performed anatomically [47, 48, 52, 65, 99].

7.2 Surgical managment

The removal of stones through the use of ERCP in patients without cholangitis can prevent the development of AP in the future, but it cannot prevent the development of biliary colic or cholecystitis. Accordingly, cholecystectomy is recommended prior to discharge in patients with mild AP and with gallstones [47, 48, 52, 65, 100–103]. Preoperative MRCP or EUS, or intraoperative cholangiography may be carried out for the selection of patients with common bile duct stones who need to be treated through an operative bile duct exploration or endoscopic sphincterotomy during a cholecystectomy [48, 52, 99]. A cholecystectomy may be avoided in ineligible elderly patients (>80 years of age), particularly if a sphincterotomy has already been performed [48, 52, 96, 97]. A cholecystectomy should be performed in patients with gallbladder sludge and AP. In patients with necrotizing biliary AP, cholecystectomies should be delayed until the active inflammation subsides and fluid collections have resolved or stabilized. If collection takes longer than 6 weeks to resolve, the cholecystectomy should be delayed until it can be performed safely [47, 48, 52, 65]. Asymptomatic pseudocysts and pancreatic and/or extrapancreatic necrosis require no surgical intervention, regardless of the size, location and/or extension. In asymptomatic patients with infected necrosis, surgical, radiological and/or endoscopic drainage should be delayed for more than 4 weeks to allow for the liquefaction of the content and the development of a fibrous wall around the necrosis (WON). Minimally invasive necrosectomy methods are preferred in symptomatic patients with infected necrosis [47, 48, 52, 84, 87]. Percutaneous drainage and/or endoscopic drainage/debridement are minimally invasive alternatives to open surgery [104].

Percutaneous CT-guided catheter drainage: The procedure is performed under local anesthesia. Depending on the size and location of the necrosis, the catheter is placed under CT guidance. Irrigation with saline every several days after insertion [105, 106]. Although percutaneous catheter drainage was used for patients who are too unstable to undergo surgical debridement, approximately one third to one half of patients can be managed with this method alone [106, 107]. The only disadvantage of this method is the risk of persistent pancreatico-cutaneous fistula [108].

Endoscopic debridement: It is performed via transgastric or transduedonal [104, 105, 109]. Cystenterostomy is created using wire-guided balloon dilators. Mechanical debridement is performed using snares, baskets, and stone retrieval balloons. Following this, a stent is placed in the cavity. The flow of necrotic contents into the stomach or duodenum is provided [109]. Minimally invasive operative approaches are preferred to open surgical necrosectomy and given lower morbidity [110].

8. Conclusion

Although new guidelines have been published, there are several knowledge gaps identified in the initial management of the AP. Risk stratification of patients with AP is important to ensure the appropriate level of care. Therefore, there is a need to develop fast, easy and practical systems that can be used in the emergency room. There is also a need to define targeted therapies in AP. Future research will enable prevention of relapse, chronicity, and cancer development, improvement of quality of life and reduction of mortality.

Acknowledgements

No funding support.

Conflict of interest

The authors declare no conflict of interest.

Author details

Rezan Karaali[1]* and Firdes Topal[2]

1 Emergency Department, Izmir Katip Celebi University Atatürk Training and Research Hospital, Izmir, Turkey

2 Gastroenterology Department, Izmir Katip Celebi University Atatürk Training and Research Hospital, Izmir, Turkey,

*Address all correspondence to: rezantahtaci@hotmail.com

References

[1] Garg SK, Sarvepalli S, Campbell JP, Obaitan I, Singh D, Bazerbahi F et al. Incidence, admission rates and predictors and economic burden of adult emergency visits for acute pancreatitis data from the national emergency department sample 2006 to 2012. J Clin Gastroenterol 2019;53(3):220-225. https://doi.org/10.1097/MCG.0000000000001030.

[2] Besinger B, Stehman CR. Pancreatitis and Cholecystitis In Tintinalli JE, Stapczynski JS, Ma OJ, Yealy DM, Meckler GD, Cline DM. editors. Tintinalli's Emergency Medicine A Comprehensive Study Guide 8th ed. Mc Graw-Hill Education; 2016. p: 517-521 ISBN: 978-0-07-180913-9.

[3] Singh VK, Bollen TL, Wu BU, et al: An assessment of the severity of interstitial pancreatitis. Clinical Gastroenterol Hepatol 2011;9(12):1098-103. https://doi.org/ 10.1016/j.cgh.2011.08.026

[4] Lankisch PG, Breuer N, Bruns A, et al: Natural history of acute pancreatitis: a long-term population-based study. Am J Gastroenterol 2009;104(11):2797-805. https://doi.org/10.1038/ajg.2009.405.

[5] Yadav D, O'Connell M, Papachristou GI: Natural history following the first attack of acute pancreatitis. Am J Gastroenterol 2012;107(7):1096-103. doi: 10.1038/ajg.2012.126.

[6] Peery AE, Dellon ES, Lund J et al. Burden of gastrointestinal diseases in the United States 2012 Update. Gastroenterology 2012;143:1179-87. https://doi.org/10.1053/j.gastro.2012.08.002.

[7] Fagenholz PJ, Fernandez-del Castillo C, Harris NS et al. Direct medical costs of acute pancreatitis hospitalizations in the United States. Pancreas 2007;35:302-7. https://doi.org/10.1097/MPA.0b013e3180cac24b.

[8] Gloor B, Müller CA, Worni M, et al. Late mortality in patients with severe acute pancreatitis. Br J Surg 2001; 88:975. https://doi.org/10.1046/j.0007-1323.2001.01813.x

[9] Mutinga M, Rosenbluth A, Tenner SM, et al. Does mortality occur early or late in acute pancreatitis? Int J Pancreatol 2000;28:91. https://doi.org/10.1385/IJGC:28:2:091.

[10] Cheon YK, Cho KB, Watkins JL, et al: Frequency and severity of post-ERCP pancreatitis correlated with extent of pancreatic ductal opacification. Gastrointest Endosc 2007;65(3):385-93. https://doi.org/10.1016/j.gie.2006.10.021.

[11] Gullo I, Migliori M, Olah A et al. Acute pancreatitis in five European countries: etiology and mortality. Pancreas 2002;24:223-7. https://doi.org/10.1097/00006676-200204000-00003.

[12] Lowenfels AB, Maisonneuve P, Sullivan T. The changing character of acute pancreatitis: epidemiology, etiology, and prognosis. Curr Gastroenterol Rep 2009;11:97-103. https://doi.org/10.1007/s11894-009-0016-4.

[13] Venneman NG, Renooij W, Rehfeld JF, et al. Small gallstones, preserved gallbladder motility, and fast crystallization are associated with pancreatitis. Hepatology 2005;41(4):738-46. https://doi.org/10.1002/hep.20616.

[14] Kristiansen L, Gronbaek M, Becker U, Tolstrup JS: Risk of pancreatitis according to alcohol drinking habits: a population-based cohort study. Am J Epidemiol

2008;168(8):932-7. https://doi.org/10.1093/aje/kwn222.

[15] Ammann RW: The naturalhistory of alcoholic chronic pancreatitis. Intern Med. 2001;40(5):368-75. https://doi.org/10.2169/internalmedicine.40.368.

[16] Takahashi T, Miao Y, Kang F, Dolai S and Gaisano HY. Susceptibility Factors and Cellular Mechanisms Underlying Alcoholic Pancreatitis. Alcohol Clin Exp Res 2020;44(4):777-789. https://doi.org/10.1111/acer.14304.

[17] Apte MV, Wilson JS, McCaughan GW, et al. Ethanol-induced alterations in messenger RNA levels correlate with glandular content of pancreatic enzymes. J Lab Clin Med 1995;125(5):634-40. PMID: 7738427.

[18] Migliori M, Manca M, Santini D, et al. Does acute alcoholic pancreatitis precede the chronic form or is the opposite true? A histological study. J Clin Gastroenterol 2004;38(3):272-5. https://doi.org/10.1097/00004836-200403000-00014.

[19] Yadav D, Pitchumoni CS. Issues in hyperlipidemic pancreatitis. J Clin Gastroenterol 2003;36(1):54-62. https://doi.org/10.1097/00004836-200301000-00016.

[20] Nawaz H, Koutroumpakis E, Easler J, et al. Elevated serum triglycerides are independently associated with persistent organ failure in acute pancreatitis. Am J Gastroenterol 2015 ;110(10):1497-503. https://doi.org/10.1038/ajg.2015.261.

[21] Wan J, He W, Zhu Y, et al. Stratified analysis and clinical significance of elevated serum triglyceride levels in early acute pancreatitis: a retrospective study. Lipids Health Dis 2017 ;16(1):124. https://doi.org/10.1186/s12944-017-0517-3.

[22] Kahaleh M, Freeman M. Prevention and management of post-endoscopic retrograde cholangio pancreatography complications. Clin Endosc 2012;45(3):305-12. https://doi.org/10.5946/ce.2012.45.3.305.

[23] Meczker A, Hanák L, Párniczky A, ET al. Analysis of 1060 Cases of Drug-Induced Acute Pancreatitis. 2020;159(5):1958-1961 DOI:https://doi.org/10.1053/j.gastro.2020.07.016.

[24] Trivedi CD, Pitchumoni CS: Drug-induced pancreatitis: an update. J Clin Gastroenterol 2005;39(8):709-16. https://doi.org/10.1097/01.mcg.0000173929.60115.b4.

[25] Badalov N, Baradarian R, Iswara K, Li J, Steinberg W, Tenner S: Drug-induced acute pancreatitis: an evidence-based review. Clin Gastroenterol Hepatol 2007;5(6):648-61; quiz 644. https://doi.org/10.1016/j.cgh.2006.11.023.

[26] Gagnon AL, Lavoie A, Frigon MP, Michaud-Herbst A, Tremblay K. A Drug-Induced Acute Pancreatitis Retrospective Study. J Gastroenterol Hepatol 2020;2020:1516493. https://doi.org/10.1155/2020/1516493.

[27] Tenner S, Steinberg WM. Acute pancreatitis In Feldman M, freidman LS, Brandt LJ editors Sleisenger and Fordtrand's gastrointestinal and liver disease: pathophihysiology, diagnosis and management book. 9th edition. Saunders-elsevier; 2010. p 959-983 ISBN: 978-1-4160-6189-2

[28] Parenti DM, Steinberg W, Kang P. Infectious causes of acute pancreatitis. Pancreas 1996;13(4):356-71. https://doi.org/10.1097/00006676-199611000-00005.

[29] Inamdar S, Benias PC, Liu Y, Sejpal DV, Satapathy SK, Trindade AJ, Prevalence, risk factors, and outcomes of hospitalized patients with COVID-19 presenting as acute pancreatitis. Gastroenterology 2020;159:2226-2228 https://doi.org/10.1053/j.gastro.2020.08.044

[30] Bokhari SMMA, Mahmood F. Case Report: Novel Coronavirus—A Potential Cause of Acute Pancreatitis?Am. J. Trop. Med. Hyg 2020;103(3):1154-1155. https://doi.org/10.4269/ajtmh.20-0568.

[31] Wilson RH, Moorehead RJ. Current management of trauma to the pancreas. Br J Surg 1991 ;78(10):1196-202. https:// doi.org/ 10.1002/bjs.1800781017.

[32] Ros E, Navarro S et al. Occult microlithiasis in idiopatic acute pancreatitis:prevention of relapses by cholecystecthomy or ursodeoxycholic acid theraphy. Gastroenterology 1991:101(6);1701-1709. https://doi.org/10.1016/0016-5085(91)90410-M

[33] Uomo G, Manes G, Ragozzino A, et al. Periampullary extraluminal duodenal diverticula and acute pancreatitis: an underestimated etiological association. Am J Gastroenterol 1996; 91:1186. PMID: 8651168

[34] Watts RA, Isenberg DA. Pancreatic disease in the autoimmune rheumatic disorders. Semin Arthritis Rheum 1989;19(3):158-65. https://doi.org/10.1016/0049-0172(89)90028-0.

[35] DiMagno MJ, Dimagno EP. Pancreas divisum does not cause pancreatitis, but associates with CFTR mutations. Am J Gastroenterol 2012;107(2):318-20. https://doi.org/ 10.1038/ajg.2011.430.

[36] SteinbergWM, Chari ST, Forsmark CE et al. Controversies in clinical pancreatology: management of acute idiopathic recurrent pancreatitis. Pancreas 2003;27(2):103-17. https://doi.org/ 10.1097/00006676-200308000-00001.

[37] Fernández-del Castillo C, Harringer W, Warshaw AL, et al. Risk factors for pancreatic cellular injury after cardiopulmonary bypass. N Engl J Med 1991;325(6):382-7. https://doi.org/ 10.1056/NEJM199108083250602.

[38] Warshaw AL, O'Hara PJ. Susceptibility of the pancreas to ischemic injury in shock. Ann Surg 1978;188(2):197-201. https://doi.org/ 10.1097/00000658-197808000-00012.

[39] Jalaly NY, Moran RA, Fargahi F, et al. An Evaluation of Factors Associated WithPathogenic PRSS1, SPINK1, CTFR, and/or CTRC Genetic Variants in Patients With Idiopathic Pancreatitis. Am J Gastroenterol 2017;112(8):1320-1329. https://doi.org/ 10.1038/ajg.2017.106.

[40] Steer ML. Pathogenesis of acute pancreatitis. Digestion 1997;58 Suppl 1:46-9. https://doi.org/ 10.1159/000201525.

[41] Halangk W, Lerch MM, Brandt-Nedelev B, et al. Role of cathepsin B in intracellular trypsinogen activation and the onset of acute pancreatitis. J ClinInvest 2000;106(6):773-81. https:// doi.org/ 10.1172/JCI9411.

[42] Prinz RA. Mechanisms of acute pancreatitis. Vascular etiology. Int J Pancreatol. 1991;9:31-8. https://doi.org/ 10.1007/BF02925576.

[43] Kingsnorth A. Role of cytokines and their inhibitors in acute pancreatitis. Gut 1997;40(1):1-4. https://doi.org/ 10.1136/gut.40.1.1.

[44] Wang GJ, Gao CF, Wei D, Wang C, Ding SQ: Acute pancreatitis: etiology and common pathogenesis. World J Gastroenterol 2009;15(12):1427-30. https://doi.org/ 10.3748/wjg.15.1427.

[45] Sah RP, Dawra RK, Saluja AK: New insights into the pathogenesis of pancreatitis. Curr Opin Gastroenterol 2013;29(5):523-30. https://doi.org/ 10.1097/MOG.0b013e328363e399.

[46] Swaroop VS, Chari ST, Clain JE. Severe acute pancreatitis. JAMA 2004; 291:2865. JAMA 2004;291(23):2865-8. https://doi.org/ 10.1001/ jama.291.23.2865.

[47] Crockett SD, Wani S, Gardner TB, Falck-Ytter Y, Barkun AY;on behalf of American Gastroenterological Association Institute Clinical Guidelines Committee American Gastroenterological Association Institute Guidelineon Initial Management of Acute Pancreatitis. Gastroenterology 2018;154:1096-1101. https://doi.org/10.1053/j.gastro.2018.01.032

[48] Tenner S, Baillie J, DeWitt J, Vege SS. American College of Gastroenterology Guideline:Management of Acute Pancreatitis. Am J Gastroenterol 2013; 108:1400-1415; https://doi.org/ 10.1038/ajg.2013.218

[49] Kiriyama S, Gabata T, Takada T, et al: New diagnostic criteria of acute pancreatitis. J Hepatobiliary Pancreat Sci 2010;17(1):24-36. https://doi.org/ 10.1007/s00534-009-0214-3.

[50] Mookadam F, Cikes M. Images in clinical medicine. Cullen's and Turner's signs. N Engl J Med 2005;353(13):1386. https://doi.org/ 10.1056/NEJMicm040796.

[51] Meyers MA, Feldberg MA, Oliphant M: Grey-Turner's sign and Cullen's sign in acute pancreatitis. Gastrointest Radiol Winter 1989;14(1):31-7. https:// doi.org/ 10.1007/BF01889150.

[52] Working Group IAP/APA Acute Pancreatitis Guidelines IAP/APA evidence-based guidelines for the management of acute pancreatitis. Pancreatology 2013;13(4 Suppl 2):e1-15. https://doi.org/ 10.1016/j.pan.2013.07.063.

[53] Yadav D, Agarwal N, Pitchumoni CS. A critical evaluation of laboratory tests in acute pancreatitis. Am J Gastroenterol 2002;97(6):1309-18. https://doi.org/ 10.1111/j.1572-0241.2002.05766.x.

[54] Winslet M, Hall C, London NJM. Relation of diagnostic serum amylase levels to aetiology and severity of acute pancreatitis. Gut 1992;33(7):982-6. doi:10.1136/gut.33.7.982.

[55] Gwozdz GP, Steinberg WM, Werner M, et al. Comparative evaluation of the diagnosis of acute pancreatitis based on serum and urine enzyme assays. Clin Chim Acta 1990;187(3):243-54. https://doi.org/10.1016/0009-8981(90)90109-6.

[56] Wu BU, Banks PA: Clinical management of patients with acute pancreatitis. Gastroenterology 2013;144(6):1272-81. https://doi.org/10.1053/j.gastro.2013.01.075.

[57] Kemppainen E, Hedström J, Puolakkainen P, et al. Increased serum trypsinogen 2 and trypsin 2-alpha 1 antitrypsin complex values identify endoscopic retrograde cholangiopancreatography induced pancreatitis with high accuracy. Gut 1997;41(5):690-5. https://doi.org/ 10.1136/gut.41.5.690.

[58] Huang QL, Qian ZX, Li H. A comparative study of the urinary trypsinogen-2, trypsinogen activation peptide, and the computed tomography severity index as early predictors of the severity of acute pancreatitis. Hepatogastroenterology 2010;57(102-103):1295-9. PMID: 21410075

[59] Mayumi T, Inui K, Maetani I, et al. Validity of the urinary trypsinogen-2 test in the diagnosis of acute pancreatitis. Pancreas 2012;41(6):869-75. https://doi.org/10.1097/MPA.0b013e3182480ab7.

[60] Tian F, Li H, Wang L, Li B et al. The diagnostic value of serum C-reactive protein, procalcitonin, interleukin-6 and lactate dehydrogenase in patients with severe acute pancreatitis. Clinica Chimica Acta 2020;510:665-670. doi:10.1016/j.cca.2020.08.029.

[61] Wang L, Qi X, Tian F, Li H et al. Diagnostic value of hematological

parameters in acute pancreatitis. Ann Palliat Med 2020 Sep;9(5):2716-2722. https://doi.org/10.21037/apm-20-160.

[62] Johnson C, L é vy P. Detection of gallstones in acute pancreatitis: when and how? Pancreatology 2010;10(1):27-32. https://doi.org/10.1159/000224147

[63] Arvanitakis M, Delhaye M, Maertelaere VD et al. Computed tomography and MRI in the assessment of acute pancreatitis. Gastroenterology. 2004;126(3):715-23. https://doi.org/10.1053/j.gastro.2003.12.006.

[64] Fleszler F, Friedenberg F, Krevsky B, Friedel D, Braitman LE: Abdominal computed tomography prolongs length of stay and is frequently unnecessary in the evaluation of acute pancreatitis. Am J Med Sci 2003;325(5):251-5. https://doi.org/10.1097/00000441-200305000-00001.

[65] Vege SS, DiMagno MJ, Forsmark CE, et al. Initial Medical Treatment of Acute Pancreatitis: American Gastroenterological Association Institute Technical Review. Gastroenterology 2018 ;154(4):1103-1139. https://doi.org/10.1053/j.gastro.2018.01.031.

[66] Banks PA, Bollen TL, Dervenis C, et al: Classification of acute pancreatitis–2012: revision of the Atlanta classification and definitions by international consensus. Gut 2013;62(1):102-11. https://doi.org/10.1136/gutjnl-2012-302779

[67] Marshall JC, Cook DJ, Christou NV et al. Multiple organ dysfunction score: a reliable descriptor of complex clinical outcome. Crit Care Med 1995;23(10):1638-52. https://doi.org/10.1097/00003246-199510000-00007.

[68] Papachristou GI, Muddana V, Yadav D, et al: Comparison of BISAP, Ranson's, APACHE-II, and CTSI scores in predicting organ failure, complications, and mortality in acute pancreatitis. Am J Gastroenterol 2010;105(2):435-41; quiz 442. https://doi.org/10.1038/ajg.2009.622.

[69] Singh VK, Wu BU, Bollen TL, et al: Early systemic inflammatory response syndrome is associated with severe acute pancreatitis. Clin Gastroenterol Hepatol 2009;7(11):1247-51. https://doi.org/10.1016/j.cgh.2009.08.012.

[70] Haydock, Mittal A, Wilms HR, et al. Fluid therapy in acute pancreatitis: anybody's guess. Ann Surg 2013;257(2):182-8. https://doi.org/10.1097/SLA.0b013e31827773ff.

[71] Zhao G, Zhang JG, Wu HS, et al. Effects of different resuscitation fluid on severe acute pancreatitis. World J Gastroenterol 2013 Apr 7;19(13):2044-52. doi: 10.3748/wjg.v19.i13.2044.

[72] Wu BU, Hwang JQ, Gardner TH, et al. Lactated Ringer's solution reduces systemic inflammation compared with saline in patients with acute pancreatitis. Clin Gastroenterol Hepatol 2011;9(8):710-717.e1. https://doi.org/10.1016/j.cgh.2011.04.026.

[73] Brown A, Orav J, Banks PA. Hemoconcentration is an early marker for organ failure and necrotizing pancreatitis. Pancreas 2000;20(4):367-72. https://doi.org/10.1097/00006676-200005000-00005.

[74] Wu BU, Johannes RS, Sun X, et al. Early changes in blood urea nitrogen predict mortality in acute pancreatitis. Gastroenterology 2009 Jul;137(1):129-35. doi: 10.1053/j.gastro.2009.03.056.

[75] Brown A, Baillargeon JD, Hughes MD, Banks PA. Can fluid resuscitation prevent pancreatic necrosis in severe acute pancreatitis? Pancreatology 2002;2(2):104-7. https://doi.org/ 10.1159/000055899.

[76] Basurto Ona X, Rigau Comas D, Urrútia G. Opioids for acute pancreatitis pain. Cochrane Database Syst Rev 2013;(7):CD009179. https://doi.org/10.1002/14651858.CD009179.pub2

[77] Helm JF, Venu RP, Geenen JE, et al. Effects of morphine on the human sphincter of Oddi. Gut 1988;29(10):1402-7. https://doi.org/10.1136/gut.29.10.1402.

[78] Yi F, Ge L, Zhao J, et al: Meta-analysis: total parenteral nutrition versus total enteral nutrition in predicted severe acute pancreatitis. Intern Med 2012;51(6):523-30. https://doi.org/10.2169/internalmedicine.51.6685.

[79] Moraes JM, Feiga GE, Chebli LA, et al: A full solid diet as the initial meal in mild acutepancreatitis is safe and result in a shorter length of hospitalization: results from a prospective, randomized, controlled, double-blind clinical trial. J Clin Gastroenterol 2010;44(7):517-522. https://doi.org/10.1097/MCG.0b013e3181c986b3

[80] Louie BE, Noseworthy T, Hailey D et al. 2004 MacLean-Mueller Prize enteral or parenteral nutrition for severe pancreatitis: a randomized controlled trial and health technology assessment. Can J Surg 2005;48(4):298-306. PMID: 16149365

[81] Casas M, Mora J, Fort E et al. Total enteral nutrition vs. total parenteral nutrition in patients with severe acute pancreatitis.Rev Esp Enferm Dig 2007;99(5):264-9. https://doi.org/10.4321/s1130-01082007000500004.

[82] Singh N, Sharma B, Sharma M et al. Evaluation of early enteral feding through nasogastric and nasojejunal tube in severe acute pancreatitis. A non-inferiority randomized controlled trial. Pancreas 2012;41(1):153-159. https://doi.org/10.1097/MPA.0b013e318221c4a8

[83] Omran M, Albalawi ZH, Tashkandi MF, Al-Ansary LA. Enteral versus parenteral nutrition for acute pancreatitis. Cochrane Database Syst Rev 2010;2010(1):CD002837. https://doi.org/ 10.1002/14651858.CD002837.pub2.

[84] Freeman MF, Werner J, van Santvoort HC et al. Interventions for necrotizing pancreatitis. Summary of a multi-disciplinary consensus conference. Pancreas 2012;41(8):1176-94. https://doi.org/10.1097/MPA.0b013e318269c660.

[85] Wittau M, Mayer B, Scheele J, Henne-Bruns D, Dellinger EP, Isenmann R: Systematic review and meta-analysis of antibiotic prophylaxis in severe acute pancreatitis. Scand J Gastroenterol 2011; 46(3):261-70. https://doi.org/10.3109/00365521.2010.531486.

[86] Lenhart DK, Balthazar EJ. MDCT of acute mild (nonnecrotizing) pancreatitis: abdominal complications and fate of fluid collections. AJR Am J Roentgenol 2008;190(3):643-9. https://doi.org/10.2214/AJR.07.2761.

[87] Clancy TE, Ashley SW. Current management of necrotizing pancreatitis. Adv Surg 2002;36:103-21. PMID: 12465548

[88] Jacobson BC, Baron TH, Adler DG, et al. ASGE guideline: The role of endoscopy in the diagnosis and the management of cystic lesions and inflammatory fluid collections of the pancreas. Gastrointest Endosc 2005;61(3):363-70. https://doi.org/10.1016/s0016-5107(04)02779-8.

[89] Seewald S, Groth S, Omar S, et al. Aggressive endoscopic therapy for pancreatic necrosis and pancreatic abscess: a new safe and effective treatment algorithm (videos). Gastrointest Endosc 2005;62(1):92-100. https://doi.org/10.1016/s0016-5107(05)00541-9.

[90] Runzi M, Niebel W, Goebell H et al. Severe acute pancreatitis: non surgical treatment of infected necrosis. Pancreas 2005;30(3):195-9. https://doi.org/10.1097/01.mpa.0000153613.17643.b3.

[91] van Brunschot S, van Grinsven J, van Santvoort HC, et al. Endoscopic or surgical step-up approach for infected necrotising pancreatitis: a multicentre randomised trial. Lancet 20186;391(10115):51-58. https://doi.org/10.1016/S0140-6736(17)32404-2.

[92] Garg PK , Sharma M , Madan K et al. Primary conservative treatment results in mortality comparable to surgery in patients with infected pancreatic necrosis. Clin Gastroenterol Hepatol 2010;8(12):1089-1094.e2. https://doi.org/10.1016/j.cgh.2010.04.011.

[93] van Santvoort HC, Besselink MG, Bakker OJ, et al. A step-up approach or open necrosectomy for necrotizing pancreatitis. N Engl J Med 2010;362(16):1491-502. https://doi.org/10.1056/NEJMoa0908821.

[94] Dellinger EP, Tellado JM, Soto NE et al. Early antibiotic treatment for severe acute necrotizing pancreatitis: a randomized, double blind, placebo controlled study. Ann Surg 2007;245(5):674-83. https://doi.org/10.1097/01.sla.0000250414.09255.84.

[95] Das S, Singh PP, Phillips A, et al. Newly diagnosed diabetes mellitus after acute pancreatitis: A systematic review and meta-analysis. Gut 2014;63(5):818-31. https://doi.org/10.1136/gutjnl-2013-305062.

[96] Schepers NJ, Hallensleben NDL, Besselink MG, et al. Urgent endoscopic retrograde cholangiopancreatography with sphincterotomy versus conservative treatment in predicted severe acute gallstone pancreatitis (APEC): a multicentre randomised controlled trial. Lancet 202018;396(10245):167-176. https://doi.org/10.1016/S0140-6736(20)30539-0.

[97] Tse F, Yuan Y. Early routine endoscopic retrograde cholangiopancreatography strategy versus early conservative management strategy in acute gallstone pancreatitis. Cochrane Database Syst Rev 2012;(5):CD009779. https://doi.org/10.1002/14651858.CD009779.pub2.

[98] Moretti A, Papi C, Aratari A et al. Is early endoscopic retrograde cholangiopancreatography useful in the management of acute biliary pancreatitis? A meta-analysis of randomized controlled trials. Dig Liver Dis2008;40(5):379-385. https://doi.org/10.1016/j.dld.2007.12.001

[99] Arguedas MR, Dupont AW, Wilcox CM. Where do ERCP, endoscopic ultrasound, magnetic resonance cholangiopancreatography, and intraoperative cholangiography ft in the management of acute biliary pancreatitis? A decision analysis model. Am J Gastroenterol 2001;96(10):2892-2899. https://doi.org/10.1016/S0002-9270(01)02806-4

[100] Larson SD, Nealson WH, Evers BM. Management of gallstone pancreatitis. Adv Surg 2006;40:265-84. https://doi.org/10.1016/j.yasu.2006.06.005.

[101] Aboulian A, Chan T, Yaghoubian A, et al. Early cholecystectomy safely decreases hospital stay in patients with mild gallstone pancreatitis: a randomized prospective study. Ann Surg 2010; 251:615. 2010;251(4):615-9. https://doi.org/ 10.1097/SLA.0b013e3181c38f1f.

[102] Falor AE, de Virgilio C, Stabile BE, et al. Early laparoscopic cholecystectomy for mild gallstone pancreatitis. Arch Surg

2012;147(11):1031-5. https://doi.org/10.1001/archsurg.2012.1473.

[103] Trna J, Vege SS, Pribramska V, et al: Lack of significant liver enzyme elevation and gallstones and/or sludge on ultrasound on day 1 of acute pancreatitis is associated with recurrence after cholecystectomy: a population-based study. Surgery 2012;151(2):199-205. https://doi.org/10.1016/j.surg.2011.07.017.

[104] Navaneethan U, Vege SS, Chari ST, Baron TH. Minimally invasive techniques in pancreatic necrosis. Pancreas 2009;38(8):867-75. https://doi.org/ 10.1097/MPA.0b013e3181b3b237.

[105] Papachristou GI, Takahashi N, Chahal P, et al. Peroral endoscopic drainage/debridement of walled-off pancreatic necrosis. Ann Surg 2007; 2007;245(6):943-51. https://doi.org/10.1097/01.sla.0000254366.19366.69.

[106] Traverso LW, Kozarek RA. Pancreatic necrosectomy: definitions and technique. J Gastrointest Surg 2005;9(3):436-9. https://doi.org/ 10.1016/j.gassur.2004.05.013.

[107] Mortelé KJ, Girshman J, Szejnfeld D, et al. CT-guided percutaneous catheter drainage of acute necrotizing pancreatitis: clinical experience and observations in patients with sterile and infected necrosis. AJR Am J Roentgenol 2009;192(1):110-6. https://doi.org/10.2214/AJR.08.1116.

[108] Gluck M, Ross A, Irani S, et al. Dual modality drainage for symptomatic walled-off pancreatic necrosis reduces length of hospitalization, radiological procedures, and number of endoscopies compared to standard percutaneous drainage. J Gastrointest Surg 2012;16(2):248-56; discussion 256-7. https://doi.org/ 10.1007/s11605-011-1759-4.

[109] Bradley EL 3rd, Howard TJ, van Sonnenberg E, Fotoohi M. Intervention in necrotizing pancreatitis: an evidence-based review of surgical and percutaneous alternatives. J Gastrointest Surg 2008;12(4):634-9. https://doi.org/ 10.1007/s11605-007-0445-z.

[110] BaronTH, DiMaio CJ , Wang AY, et al. American Gastroenterological Association Clinical Practice Update: Management of Pancreatic Necrosis Gastroenterology 2020;158(1):67-75.e1. https://doi.org/ 10.1053/j.gastro.2019.07.064.

Chapter 2

Necrotizing Pancreatitis: Step Up Approach

Betsabé Reyes, Javier Padilla, Pilar Elena González and Pablo Sanz

Abstract

Acute pancreatitis (AP) is a inflamatory condition of the pancreatic gland with or without involvement of peripancreatic tissues and distant organs. The incidence of AP is 20–35 cases per 100,000 inhabitants per year, with an overall mortality of 2–10%. In recent decades the incidence of AP has increased globally. Most cases follow a mild, self-limiting course, but 10–20% of patients develop a severe form with systemic and local life-threatening complications of pancreatic and peripancreatic necrosis come about 20–40% of patient with severe AP and aggravate organ functions. The traditional approach to the treatment of necrotizing pancreatitis with secondary infection of necrotic tissue is open necrosectomy to remove the infected necrotic tissue. But this is associated with high rates of complications, death and pancreatic insufficiency. The benefits of sequential treatment in cases of infected necrosis ("Step an approach") compared to traditional open necrosectomy, showing less morbidity and lower costs. The sequential treatment is an alternative to open necrosectomy, including percutaneous drainage, endoscopic (transgastric) drainage, and minimally invasive retroperitoneal necrosectomy. With this approach, up to 35% of patients can be treated only with drainage, to avoid necrosectomy and to reduce the percentage of complications. In this chapter we present the step-by-step approach.

Keywords: necrotizing pancreatitis, step up approach, acute pancreatitis, percutaneous, endoscopic, necrosectomy

1. Introduction

Acute pancreatitis (AP) is a inflamatory condition of the pancreatic gland with or without involvement of peripancreatic tissues and distant organs [1]. The incidence of AP is 20–35 cases per 100,000 inhabitants per year, with an overall mortality of 2–10%. In recent decades the incidence of AP has increased globally and is expected to increase even more. The most common cause is biliary lithiasis, which accounts for about 40–50%. The alcohol, predominantly in males, is the second most common cause, at over 30% and 10–25% the cause is unknown.

Most cases follow a mild, self-limiting course, but 10–20% of patients develop a severe form with systemic and local life-threatening complications of pancreatic and peripancreatic necrosis come about 20–40% of patient with severe AP and aggravate organ functions [2–6]. Infected necrotic tissue is defined as a gram positive of pancreatic or peripancreatic necrotic tissue obtained by means of fine-needle aspiration or from the first drainage procedure or operation, or the presence of gas in the fluid collection on contrast-enhanced computer tomography (CT). Suspected infected necrosis is defined as persistent sepsis or progressive clinical deterioration in the intensive care unit without documentation of infected necrosis. Failure of one or more organs occurs in 40% of these patients with pancreatic necrosis and on rare occasions it can also occur in cases without necrosis. Mortality amounts to 30% when infection of the pancreatic and/or peripancreatic necrosis is present [7].

The traditional approach to the treatment of necrotizing pancreatitis with secondary infection of necrotic tissue is open necrosectomy to remove the infected necrotic tissue. But this is associated with high rates of complications, death and pancreatic insufficiency. The studies show that death rates from open pancreatic necrosectomy are between 10–40% [8–10]. The management of AP has evolved greatly in recent years thanks to a better understanding of pathophysiology, the improvement of the therapeutic arsenal of intensive care units, nutritional support, conventional and interventional radiology techniques and surgical treatment. Recently, a randomized trial called "PANTER" very well designed study by the Dutch Pancreatitis Study Group, demonstrated the benefits of sequential treatment in cases of infected necrosis ("Step an approach") compared to traditional open necrosectomy, showing less morbidity and lower costs [7]. The sequential treatment is an alternative to open necrosectomy, less invasive techniques, including percutaneous drainage, endoscopic (transgastric) drainage, and minimally invasive retroperitoneal necrosectomy. The importance of step up approach is that the first step is percutaneous or endoscopic drainage of the collection of infected fluid to mitigate sepsis and this step may postpone or even obviate surgical necrosectomy. If the drainage does not take to clinical recovery, the next step is minimally invasive retroperitoneal necrosectomy. With this approach, up to 35% of patients can be treated only with drainage, to avoid necrosectomy and to reduce the percentage of complications [7].

2. Clasification acute necrotizing pancreatitis

Before to describe the management of infected necrosis, we need to know the classification of acute pancreatitis [11, 12].

The severity of acute pancreatitis can be defined as mild, moderately severe, or severe according to the revised Atlanta classification (**Table 1**).

- Mild acute pancreatitis: absence of organ failure or local and/or systemic complications.

- Moderate acute pancreatitis: organ failure, and/or transient local or systemic complications that resolve within 48 hours maximum. Mortality in this group is less than 8%.

Mild acute pancreatitis	absence of OF or local and/or systemic complications
Moderate acute pancreatitis	OF and/or transient local or systemic complications <48 hours
Severe acute pancreatitis	OF and/or transient local or systemic complications >48 hours
Potentially severe acute pancreatitis	OF or warning pancreatic sign (**Table 2**)

Table 1.
Clinical classification of pancreatitis (OF: Organ failure).

- Severe acute pancreatitis: continued organic failure over 48 hours accompanied by local and/or systemic complications. Mortality in this group is 36–50%.

- Potentially severe acute pancreatitis: organ failure or a warning sign at the beginning of its evolution (**Table 2**), and therefore requires closer monitoring, to anticipate the development of transitory, persistent organ failure or pancreatic infection. The need to detect and treat patients who are developing organ failure with invasive resuscitation measures as early as possible has been demonstrated with a strong degree of recommendation and a high level of evidence.

There is another classification of AP severity that adds another step to the severity of these processes: Acute critical pancreatitis, in which persistent organ failure (OF) coexists with necrosis infection, described in 2012 by Petrov et al.

Classification according to radiological characteristics according to the Atlanta Classification:

- Interstitial o edematous pancreatitis: the pancreas is enlargement due to inflammation or edema. The pancreatic parenchyma shows homogeneous enhancement, and the peripancreatic fat usually shows some inflammatory changes. Besides there may be some peripancreatic fluid. The clinical symptoms of interstitial o edematous pancreatitis usually resolve within the first week.

- Necrotising pancreatitis: about 5–10% of patients develop necrosis of the pancreatic parenchyma, the peripancreatic tissue or both. Necrotising pancreatitis shows necrosis involving the pancreas and peripancreatic tissues and less commonly as necrosis of only the peripancreatic tissue or pancreatic parenchyma alone. The natural history of pancreatic and peripancreatic necrosis is variable, because it may remain solid or liquefy, remain sterile or become infected, persist or disappear over time. The presence of infection can be proved by extraluminal gas in the pancreatic and/or peripancreatic tissues or when percutaneous fine-needle aspiration is positive for bacteria and/or fungi on Gram.

Local complications of acute pancreatitis:

- Acute peripancreatic liquid collection: presence of peripancreatic liquid in the context of edematous interstitial pancreatitis. It occurs in the first 4 weeks

Characteristics of patient	Analitics parameters	Radiological Features	Forecast scales
Age > 50 years	BUN >20 mg/dl	Pleural Effusion	APACHE II >2
BMI < 30	Hematocrit >44%	Pancreatic collections or peritoneal free liquid.	Ranson-Glasgow >3
Deteriorate state of mind	Procalcitonin >0.5 ng/ml in the first 48 hours		
Comorbidity	Reactive C protein >150 mgl, or progressive elevation in 48 hours)		
Abdominal defense	Elevated Creatinine		

Table 2.
Warning pancreatic sign (BMI: Body mass index, BUN: Blood urea nitrogen).

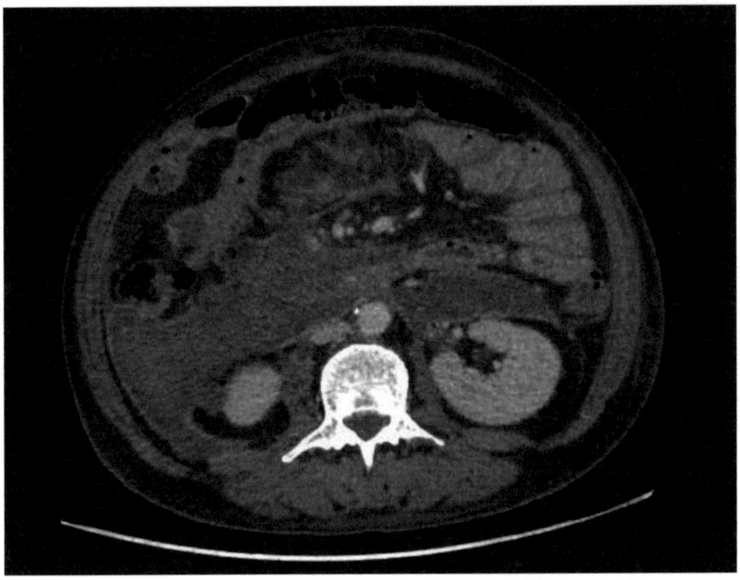

Figure 1.
In the CT scan image we can see acute pancreatic collection without radiological signs of infection.

and is characterized by the appearance of homogeneous fluid adjacent to the pancreas and its fascial planes without the presence of a wall.

- Pancreatic pseudocyst: well-defined collection with a wall formed without a solid component that occurs after 4 weeks of oedematous interstitial pancreatitis.

- Acute necrotic collection: collection with a solid and liquid component that appears in the context of necrotizing pancreatitis and can affect the pancreas and surrounding tissues. It has no wall (**Figure 1**).

- Encapsulated pancreatic necrosis (Walled-off necrosis): is an acute necrotic collection, mature, encapsulated with a well-defined inflammatory wall, and which appears 4 weeks after the onset of necrotic pancreatitis. It is heterogeneous and can affect peripancreatic tissues.

3. Infected pancreatic necrosis

The most important consideration in treating local complications is to demonstrate the presence of infection.

Because the majority of patients with sterile pancreatic or peripancreatic necrosis can be treated conservatively, regardless of the size and extension of the collections.

Drainage in a sterile collection can produce iatrogenic infection, worsening the patient's prognosis. Could only be an alternative in those patients with persistent symptoms such as abdominal pain, duodenal obstruction or jaundice [13, 14].

Necrosis infection usually occurs within 2–3 weeks of the onset of BP. Successive CT scans should be performed according to the evolution of the patient and not in a programmed way. Early onset is rare, and should be suspected if SIRS persists or recurs after 10 days-2 weeks [15]. Therefore, the suspicion of infection will be made according to the bad evolution of the patient: fever, increase of leukocytes, elevation of

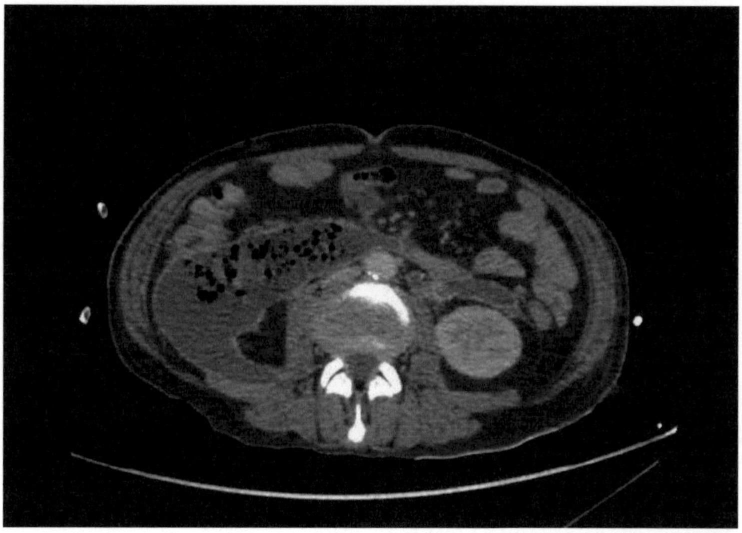

Figure 2.
CT scan image showing radiological signs of pancreatic necrosis due to the presence of gas in the acute necrotic collection.

PCR and/or procalcitonin, sudden resurgence or worsening of FO. This clinical evolution can be given by sterile necrosis, and it is often a challenge to differentiate whether we are dealing with an infected necrosis or not. Given this scenario, CT has high sensitivity to detect signs of infection (gas in the collection only appears in 12–22% of infected cases (**Figure 2**). However the signs of infection are usually sufficient to diagnose a secondary infection of pancreatic or peripancreatic necrosis. In case of diagnostic uncertainty, a positive gram stain or culture of the necrotic collection, obtained by transabdominal fine needle aspiration, may be necessary. However, the disadvantage of fine needle aspiration in this scenario is the false negative rate of 25% [16].

4. Management off infection of pancreatic necrosis

We present the management of acute pancreatitis with signs of infected necrosis. For this we will describe each of the therapeutic options in the philosophy of step up approach (Algorithm 1).

4.1 Antibiotic therapy

The first step is the administration of broad- spectrum antibiotic therapy [16]. The germs most involved are *E. coli*, *Enterobacter cloacae*, *Enterococcus faecalis* and Bacteriodes fragilis, and the antibiotic of choice for empirical treatment in these cases would be carbapenemics. In cases of allergy, quinolones would be used.

Recommended empirical therapy:

- Meropenem: 1 gr. e.v. every 8 hours
- Moxifloxacin: 400 mg e.v. every 24 hours

Once the final result of the cultivation is obtained, the anti-biotherapy will be adapted. A small proportion of patients can be managed with supportive care and antibiotics alone, without the need for additional invasive interventions [17].

4.2 The step-up approach

Open surgery in the treatment of infected pancreatic necrosis has been replaced by the minimally invasive approach. The multi-centre randomized clinical trial PANTER [18] showed that step up approach treatment of necrotising pancreatitis reduces patient mortality, multiorgan failure, costs and late surgical complications. The step-up approach consists of percutaneous catheter drainage or endoscopic transluminal drainage, followed by minimally invasive necrosectomy only when clinically required, is the current standard treatment [19].

4.2.1 Percutaneous catheter drainage

Secondary infection of pancreatic or peripancreatic necrosis can occur in the first 3 weeks after onset of disease, and long-term administration of antibiotics might lead to increased incidence of fungal infections and antibiotic resistance [15, 20]. The benefit of early drainage has been demonstrated, although its indication has to be established after confirmation of infection, otherwise we could be infecting a sterile collection. The ideal percutaneous drainage would be via the retroperitoneal route and on the left side, which would facilitate subsequent minimally invasive surgical access if necessary. Current evidence shows that 35% of patients treated with percutaneous drainage in this phase will not require additional surgical necrosectomy and that up to 50% in series where a progressive increase in the diameter of the drainage catheter is used [19]. Once the radiological drainage was carried out, the therapeutic sequence would be as follows:

if poor evolution persists after 48 hours and the patient's conditions permit it, a new drainage with a larger diameter would be attempted.

if the poor clinical condition is maintained, despite the use of larger drains, surgical drainage should be carried out.

The current tendency is to be as non-invasive as possible. Several techniques have been described that will be developed in our service gradually, such as video assisted retroperitoneal access that presents significantly lower rates of abdominal complications than the most classic techniques. This technique uses radiological drainage as a guide to the collection, hence the importance of placing it on the left side as long as possible (**Figure 3**).

After 4 weeks, in addition to percutaneous radiological drainage in case of infection as mentioned above, endoscopic drainage could be evaluated. Generally, at this stage an inflammatory wall would already be formed consistent enough to withstand transgastic endoscopic drainage (walled-off necrosis).

4.2.2 Transgastric endoscopic drainage

The step-up approach can be done both surgically and endoscopically. The two different approaches have been compared with each other in two randomized trials. The first is the TENSION trial that concluded that the endoscopic step-up approach was not superior to the surgical step-up approach in reducing major complications or death but the rate of pancreatic fistulas and length of hospital stay were lower in the endoscopy group [21]. The second trial is MISER [22] randomizade controlled trial showed that an endoscopic transluminal approach for infected necrotizing pancreatitis, compared with minimally invasive surgery, significantly reduced major complications, lowered costs, and increased quality of life.

In short, the endoscopic staggered approach has become the approach of choice according to recent studies for the management of infected necrotizing pancreatitis [23–27]. However it could not be feasible in all patients. It depends

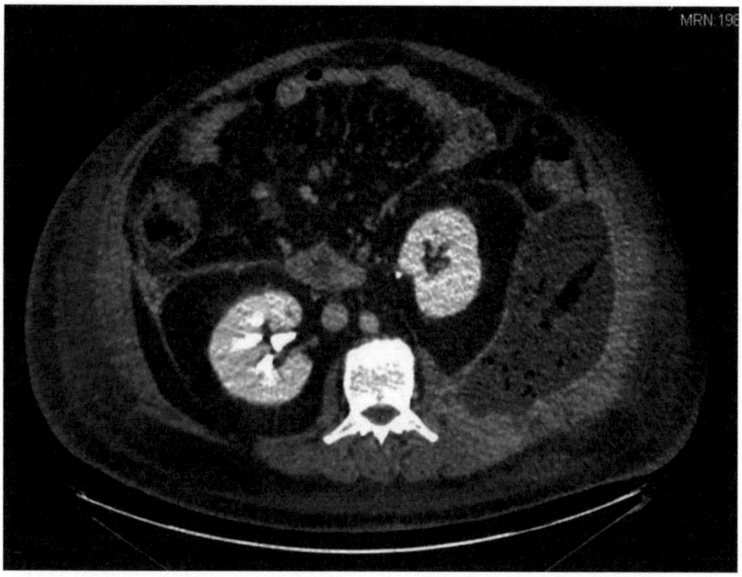

Figure 3.
CT scan image showing left retroperitoneal collection with easy access for percutaneous drainage. And it will allow a retroperitoneal laparoscopic approach.

on the anatomical location of the infected necrotic collections, availability of technique and experience of the center and trained personnel (**Figure 4**). The option of combined endoscopic transluminal and percutaneous catheter drainage, which is also known as dual-modality drainage, should not be overlooked in patients with large collections extending into the paracolic gutters or the pelvic region.

Currently, the stents placed between gastric light and the infected collection are metallic (**Figure 5**). They were created in 2011 and replaced with plastic stents. These stents provide wider light that allows better drainage and facilitates transluminal necrosectomy. The best available evidence comes from a randomized trial

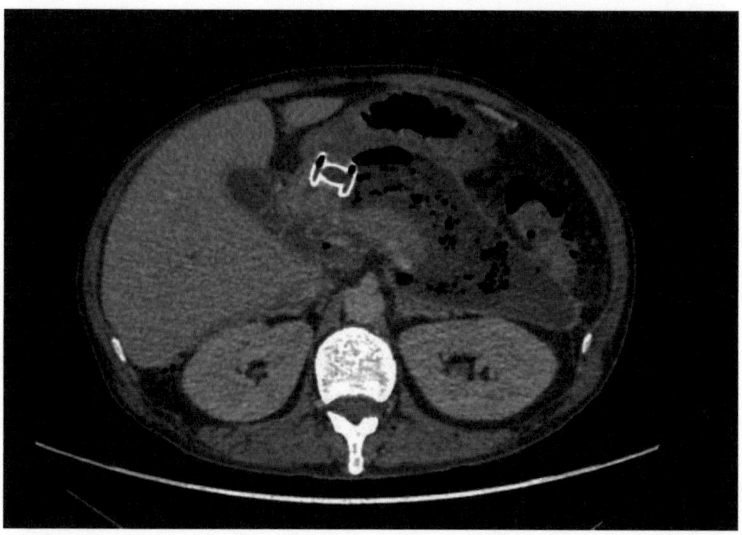

Figure 4.
CT scan image showing infected acute necrotic collection of retrogastric location. We can see metallic stent drainage inside the collection.

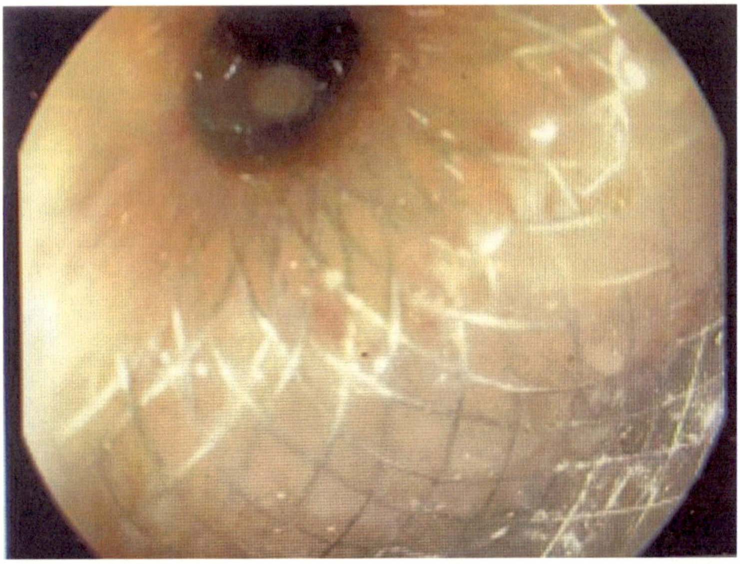

Figure 5.
Endoscopy image showing metallic stent that communicates the gastric camera and the acute necrotic collection.

that compared the efficacy of metal and plastic stents in the drainage of infected pancreatic necrosis. The study found no differences in the median number of procedures, readmissions, and length of hospital stay [28]. Although endoscopic treatment with metal stents was associated with higher procedure costs. In addition, adverse effects such as stent migration were observed. Therefore, the latest consensus guidelines recommend metal stents or double pigtail plastic stents for endoscopic transluminal drainage and removal after 4 weeks to minimize the risks of complications [28, 29].

4.2.3 Surgical necrosectomy

Between 23–47% of patients will improve only with percutaneous or endoscopic drainage. But in those patients with persistent disease, surgery is the next step [18, 30, 31]. Objectives of surgical debridement are to control the source of infection and reduce the burden of necrosis, while minimizing the proinflammatory damage of the intervention itself on the weakened patient. The current trend is to be as non-invasive as possible. We will start with a videoassisted retroperitoneal approach and if it is not enough we will perform necrosectomy by open approach [32].

4.2.3.1 Video assited retroperitoneal debridement (VARD) in infected necrotizing pancreatitis

Several techniques have been described, such as video assisted retroperitoneal access that presents significantly lower rates of abdominal complications than the most classic techniques. This technique uses radiological drainage as a guide to the collection, hence the importance of placing it on the left side as long as possible. The tract formed by the anterior drainage is used to access the retroperitoneal space for intracavitary videoassisted necrosectomy (**Figure 6**). Traditional laparoscopic instruments are used under direct vision (**Figures** 7 and **8**). We can leave well-positioned drains that allow washing. The process may be repeated if necessary to remove the infected pancreatic necrosis. It should be noted that the VARD approach is more effective in treating central to left parietocolic infected pancreatic necrosis. However, it will be more difficult to access the necrosis located to the right of the mesenteric vessels [32] (**Figure 9**).

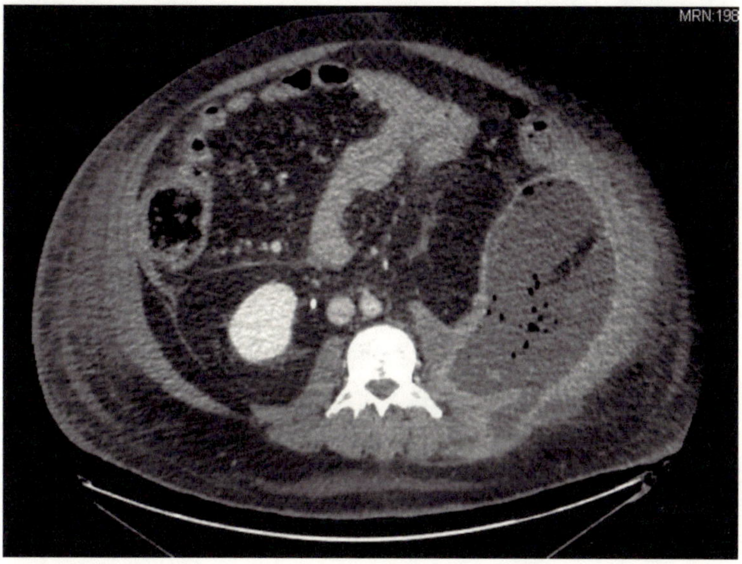

Figure 6.
CT scan image showing infected acute necrotic collection on the left flank. It allows a percutaneous drainage approach and subsequent laparoscopic retroperitoneal access.

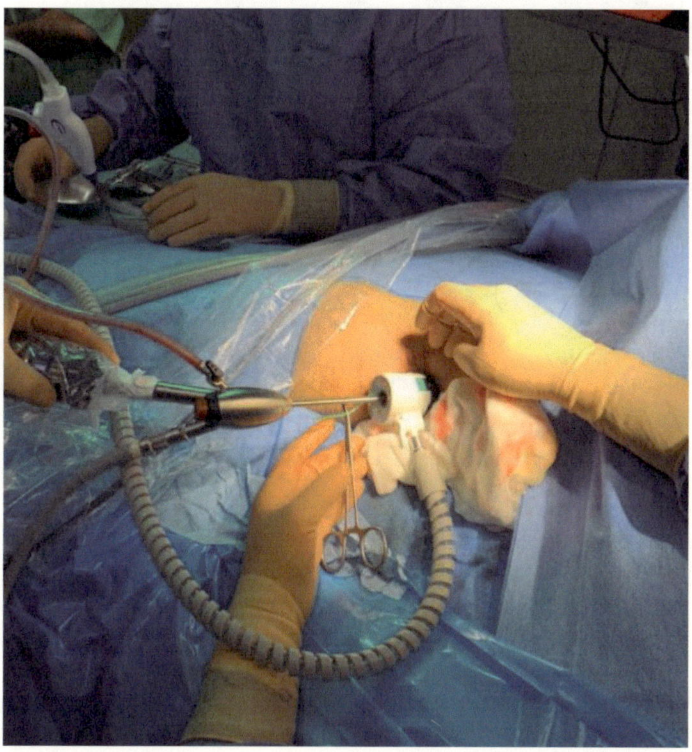

Figure 7.
Using left retroperitoneal percutaneous drainage as a guide, we can access it by minimally invasive approach. We observed laparoscopic trócar through which we introduced camera, vacuum cleaner and laparoscopic tweezers.

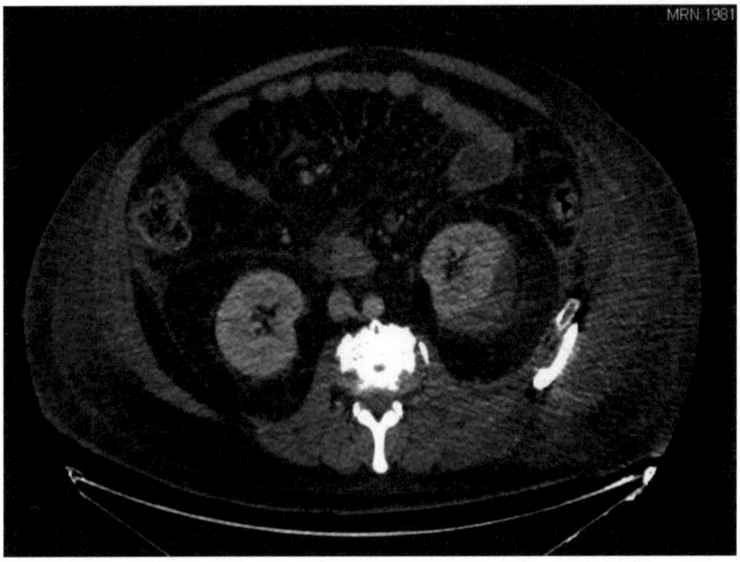

Figure 8.
Image of CT scan that objective retroperitoneal necrotic collection with drainage inside placed by laparoscopic retroperitoneal access.

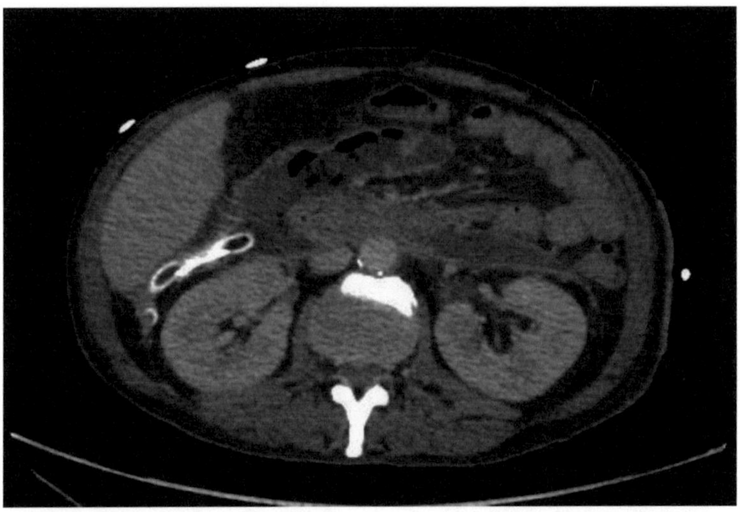

Figure 9.
CT scan showing surgical drainage on the right flank by laparoscopic retroperitoneal access.

4.2.3.2 Surgical transgastric debridement

The concept is similar to endoscopic trasngastic drainage. It can be performed by open or laparoscopic approach. An anterior gastrostomy is required to access the posterior face of the stomach and then the infected cavity. It is especially useful in central collections that do not affect the flanks (**Figure 10**). It is advisable to leave a drain inside the cavity for washing. There are studies of small sample size that demonstrate the efficacy of the technique with low morbidity [33–35].

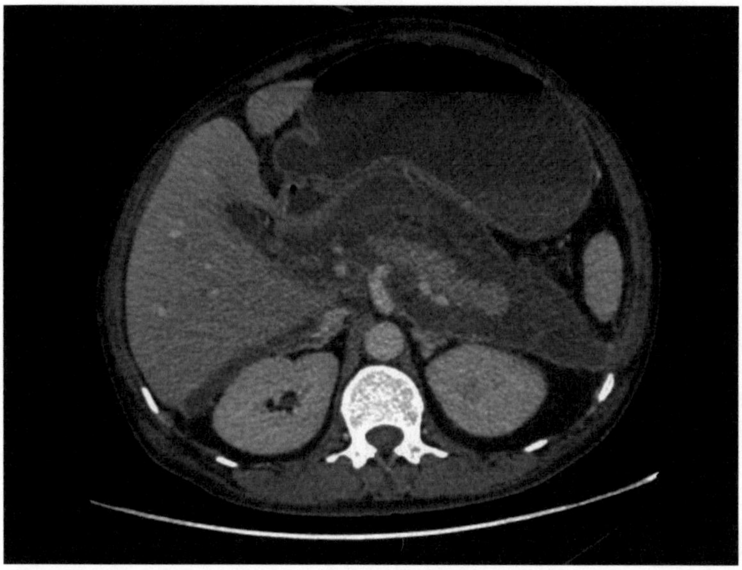

Figure 10.
CT scan image showing collection near the gastric posterior wall that would allow a transgastic approach.

4.2.3.3 Open surgical necrosectomy

If these methods are unable to control the infectious condition, the patient's deterioration, despite good drainage, including minimally invasive surgical drainage, would be indicated to the open surgical approach. The mortality of patients with infected necrosis is greater than 30%, as we have commented, the delay in surgery as much as possible will be more beneficial for the patient in terms of mortality and morbidity. Early debridement, and especially sterile necrosis, leads to a significant increase in mortality. Therefore, these techniques are reserved when everything else has not been enough [36–37]. We have widely described open necrosectomy techniques. None of them has been shown to be clearly superior to the other due to the lack of randomized studies, but the ones that offer the best results are:

- Open surgical necrosectomy with closed packing: described by A.L. Warshaw, with lower mortality rates than the other techniques (10%) and that would be indicated in limited necrosis.

- Open surgical necrosectomy with closed postoperative lavage: in case of more extensive necrosis. The recommended wash would be 12–24 liters every 24 hours with potassium-free dialysis fluid.

- Open surgical necrosectomy with open packing: it is the technique with the highest morbidity-mortality, but it would be indicated in cases with more extensive necrosis that exceed the colon.

Vacuum Assisted Closure therapy will be used as a temporary closure in cases where closure of the abdominal pare is impossible or in cases of abdominal compartment syndrome.

Current comparative studies, with the exception of randomized trials [18], should be interpreted with caution, given the severity of the often higher disease in

	Ramson	Glasgow
on admission	age > 55 yerars	age > 55 years
	white blood cell count>16.000 mm3	blood glucose>10 mmol/l
	blood glucose >200 mg %	LDH > 600 UI/l
	LDH > 400 UI/l	AST > 100 UI/l
	AST > 200 UI/l	serum urea>16 mmol/l
		Arterial PaO2 < 60%
		serum Calcium<8 mg/dl
		serum albumin<3,2 mg/l
		white blood cell count>15.000 mm3
within 48 hours	hematocrit fall>10%	
	blood urea nitrogen rise >5 mg%	
	Arterial PaO2 < 60 mmHg	
	base deficit>4 mEq/l	
	fluid sequestration >6 liters	
	serum calcium<8 mg%	

Table 3.
Ramson and Glasgow prognostic scale.

patients undergoing open debridement. Open debridement is indicated in patients with a high necrosis load that is diffusely distributed throughout the abdomen and that do not respond to staggered handling [32].

RAMSON: Prognostic scale in acute pancreatitis (**Table 3**).

GLASGOW: Prognostic scale in acute pancreatitis (**Table 3**).

Zero to do criteria met indicates mild pancreatitis; 3 or more criteria severe pancreatitis.

According to the number of criteria the rate of mortality is: 0–2 mortality >2%; 3–5 mortality 10–20%; 6–7 mortality 50–60%; > 7 mortality 70–90%.

5. Conclusions

Patients with diagnosis of acute necrotizing pancreatitis should be treated in centers with high experience by specialists in pancreatic surgery, endoscopists and radiologist experienced. It is essential the presence of a team of intensive doctors or anesthesiologists especially in the first weeks of evolution. Despite these measures the morbidity and mortality in these patients is still high, so we must try to reduce it with a correct management and applying the "step up approach". The sequential treatment is an alternative to open necrosectomy, including percutaneous drainage, endoscopic (transgastric) drainage, and minimally invasive retroperitoneal necrosectomy. With this approach, up to 35% of patients can be treated only with drainage, to avoid necrosectomy and to reduce the percentage of complications.

Acknowledgements

Our thanks to the Biliopancreatic Surgery Unit that through effort and study have created a protocol for the management of severe pancreatitis. The team is made up of expert pancreatic surgeons, intensivist physicians, anesthesiologists, endoscopists with experience in echoendoscopy and radiologists specializing in the abdomen. Together we will continue to train for the good of our patients.

Conflict of interest

The authors declare no conflict of interest.

Notes/thanks/other declarations

None

Appendices and nomenclature

Algorithm 1. Management of acute pancreatitis with infected pancreatic necrosis.

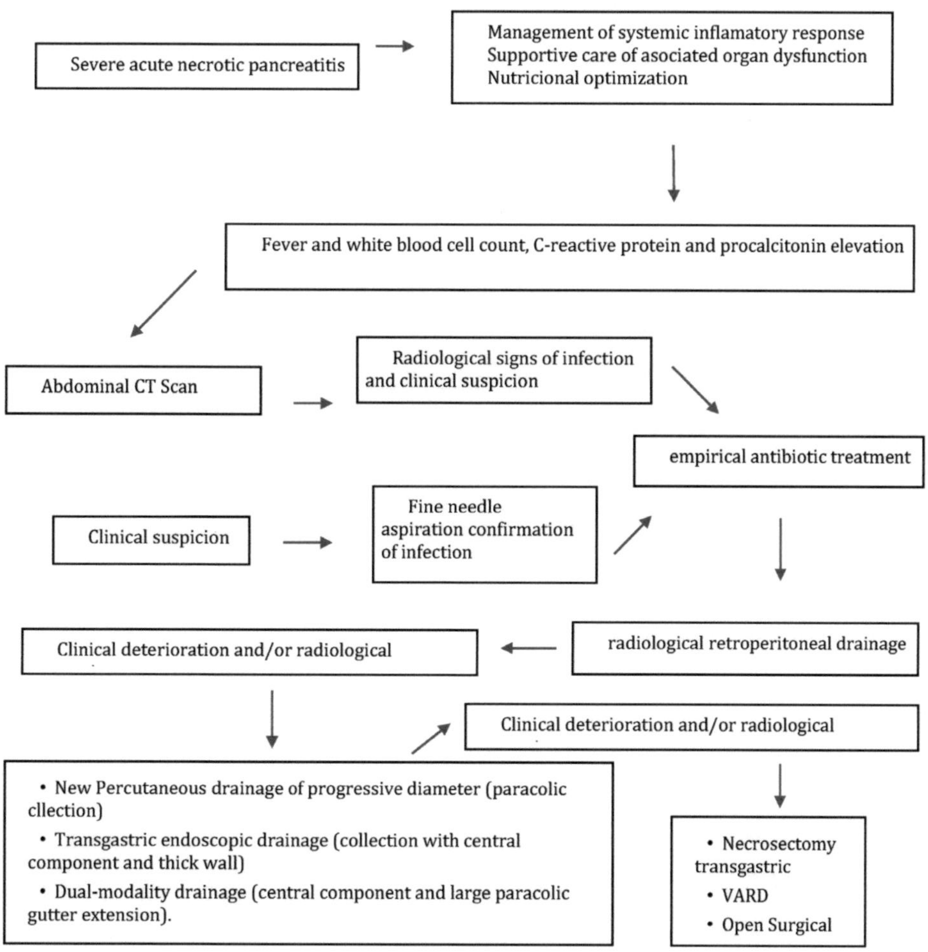

AP	acute pancreatitis
Step an approach:	staggered approach
CT	computer tomography
OF	organ failure
BMI	body mass index
BUN	blood urea nitrogen
LDH	lactate dehydrogenase
AST	aaspartate ainotranferase
PaO2	blood pressure from oxygen
VARD	video assited retroperitoneal debridement
APACHE	acute physiology and cronic health evaluation (**Figure 11**).

PHYSIOLOGIC VARIABLE	HIGH ABNORMAL RANGE						LOW ABNORMAL RANGE		
	+4	+3	+2	+1	0	+1	+2	+3	+4
TEMPERATURE — rectal (°C)	≥41°	39°-40.9°		38.5°-38.9°	36°-38.4°	34°-35.9°	32°-33.9°	30°-31.9°	≤29.9°
MEAN ARTERIAL PRESSURE — mm Hg	≥160	130-159	110-129		70-109		50-69		≤49
HEART RATE (ventricular response)	≥180	140-179	110-139		70-109		55-69	40-54	≤39
RESPIRATORY RATE — (non-ventilated or ventilated)	≥50	35-49		25-34	12-24	10-11	6-9		≤5
OXYGENATION: A-aDO$_2$ or PaO$_2$ (mm Hg) a. FIO$_2$ ≥0.5 record A-aDO$_2$	≥500	350-499	200-349		<200				
b. FIO$_2$ <0.5 record only PaO$_2$					PO$_2$ >70	PO$_2$ 61-70		PO$_2$ 55-60	PO$_2$ <55
ARTERIAL pH	≥7.7	7.6-7.69		7.5-7.59	7.33-7.49		7.25-7.32	7.15-7.24	<7.15
SERUM SODIUM (mMol/L)	≥180	160-179	155-159	150-154	130-149		120-129	111-119	≤110
SERUM POTASSIUM (mMol/L)	≥7	6-6.9		5.5-5.9	3.5-5.4	3-3.4	2.5-2.9		<2.5
SERUM CREATININE (mg/100 ml) (Double point score for **acute** renal failure)	≥3.5	2-3.4	1.5-1.9		0.6-1.4		<0.6		
HEMATOCRIT (%)	≥60		50-59.9	46-49.9	30-45.9		20-29.9		<20
WHITE BLOOD COUNT (total/mm3) (in 1,000s)	≥40		20-39.9	15-19.9	3-14.9		1-2.9		<1
GLASGOW COMA SCORE (GCS): Score = 15 minus actual GCS									
[A] Total ACUTE PHYSIOLOGY SCORE (APS): Sum of the 12 individual variable points									
Serum HCO$_3$ (venous-mMol/L) [Not preferred, use if no ABGs]	≥52	41-51.9		32-40.9	22-31.9		18-21.9	15-17.9	<15

[B] **AGE POINTS:**
Assign points to age as follows:

AGE(yrs)	Points
≤44	0
45-54	2
55-64	3
65-74	5
≥75	6

[C] **CHRONIC HEALTH POINTS**
If the patient has a history of severe organ system insufficiency or is immuno-compromised assign points as follows:
a. for nonoperative or emergency postoperative patients — 5 points
or
b. for elective postoperative patients — 2 points

DEFINITIONS
Organ Insufficiency or immuno-compromised state must have been evident **prior** to this hospital admission and conform to the following criteria:

LIVER: Biopsy proven cirrhosis and documented portal hypertension; episodes of past upper GI bleeding attributed to portal hypertension; or prior episodes of hepatic failure/encephalopathy/coma.

CARDIOVASCULAR: New York Heart Association Class IV.

RESPIRATORY: Chronic restrictive, obstructive, or vascular disease resulting in severe exercise restriction, i.e., unable to climb stairs or perform household duties; or documented chronic hypoxia, hypercapnia, secondary polycythemia, severe pulmonary hypertension (>40mmHg), or respirator dependency.

RENAL: Receiving chronic dialysis.

IMMUNO-COMPROMISED: The patient has received therapy that suppresses resistance to infection, e.g., immuno-suppression, chemotherapy, radiation, long term or recent high dose steroids, or has a disease that is sufficiently advanced to suppress resistance to infection, e.g., leukemia, lymphoma, AIDS.

APACHE II SCORE
Sum of [A] + [B] + [C]
[A] APS points
[B] Age points
[C] Chronic Health points
Total APACHE II

Figure 11.
APACHE SCALE. Health care Financ rev. 1984 Nov; 1984(Suppl): 91–105.

Author details

Betsabé Reyes*, Javier Padilla, Pilar Elena González and Pablo Sanz
Department of Surgery, Hospital Nuestra Señora de la Candelaria, Tenerife, Spain

*Address all correspondence to: reyescorreabetsabe@gmail.com

References

[1] Ari Leppäniemi , Matti Tolonen , Antonio Tarasconi Emiliano Gamberini et al. . 2019 WSES guidelines for the management of severe acute pancreatitis. Leppäniemi et al. World Journal of Emergency Surgery (2019) 14:27.

[2] Banks PA, Freeman ML. Practice guide- lines in acute pancreatitis. Am J Gastro- enterol 2006;101:2379-400.

[3] Whitcomb DC. Acute pancreatitis. N Engl J Med 2006;354:2142-50.

[4] Uhl W, Warshaw A, Imrie C, et al. IAP guidelines for the surgical management of acute pancreatitis. Pancreatology 2002;2: 565-73.

[5] Nathens AB, Curtis JR, Beale RJ, et al. Management of the critically ill patient with severe acute pancreatitis. Crit Care Med 2004;32:2524-36.

[6] Forsmark CE, Baillie J, AGA Institute Clinical Practice and Economics Commit- tee, A[GA Institute Governing Board. AGA Institute technical review on acute pan- creatitis. Gastroenterology2007;132:2022-44.

[7] Hjalmar C. van Santvoort, M.D., Marc G. Besselink, M.D., Ph.D., Olaf J. Bakker, M.D et al , for the Dutch Pancreatitis Study Group*. A Step-up Approach or Open Necrosectomy for Necrotizing Pancreatitis. N Engl J Med 2010;362:1491-502.

[8] Beger HG, Büchler M, Bittner R, Oet- tinger W, Block S, Nevalainen T. Necro- sectomy and postoperative local lavage in patients with necrotizing pancreatitis: re- sults of a prospective clinical trial. World J Surg 1988;12:255-62.

[9] Traverso LW, Kozarek RA. Pancreatic necrosectomy: definitions and technique. J Gastrointest Surg 2005;9:436-9.

[10] Lotte Boxhoorn, Rogier P Voermans, Stefan A Bouwense, Marco J Bruno, Robert C Verdonk, Marja A Boermeester, Hjalmar C van Santvoort, Marc G Besselink. Acute pancreatitis. Lancet, 2020 Sep 5;396(10252):726-734. doi: 10.1016/S0140-6736(20)31310-6.

[11] Classification of acute pancreatitis 2012: revision of the Atlanta classification and definitions by international consensus. Banks PA, Bollen TL, Dervenis C et al. Gut 2013; 62: 102-111

[12] Dellinger EP, Forsmark CE, Layer P, et al. Determinant-based classification of acute pancreatitis severity: an international multidisciplinary consultation. Ann Surg 2012; 256: 875-80

[13] Walser EM, Nealon WH, Marroquin S, Raza S, Hernandez JA, Vasek J. Sterile fluid collections in acute pancreatitis: catheter drainage versus simple aspiration. Cardiovasc Intervent Radiol 2006; 29: 102-07.

[14] Zerem E, Imamovic G, Omerović S, Imširović B. Randomized controlled trial on sterile fluid collections management in acute pancreatitis: should they be removed? Surg Endosc 2009; 23: 2770-77.

[15] Van Grinsven J, van Brunschot S, van Baal MC, et al. Natural history of gas configurations and encapsulation in necrotic collections during necrotizing pancreatitis. J Gastrointest Surg 2018; 22: 1557-64.

[16] Working Group IAP/APA acute pancreatitis guidelines. IAP/APA evidence-based guidelines for the management of acute pancreatitis. Pancreatology 2013; 13: e1-15.

[17] van Santvoort HC, Bakker OJ, Bollen TL, et al. A conservative and minimally invasive approach to necrotizing pancreatitis improves

outcome. Gastroenterology 2011; 141: 1254-63.

[18] van Santvoort HC, Besselink MG, Bakker OJ, et al. A step-up approach or open necrosectomy for necrotizing pancreatitis. N Engl J Med 2010; 362: 1491-502

[19] van Grinsven J, van Brunschot S, Bakker OJ, et al. Diagnostic strategy and timing of intervention in infected necrotizing pancreatitis: an international expert survey and case vignette study. HPB (Oxford) 2016; 18: 49-56.

[20] Besselink MG, van Santvoort HC, Boermeester MA, et al. Timing and impact of infections in acute pancreatitis. Br J Surg 2009; 96: 267-73.

[21] van Brunschot S, van Grinsven J, van Santvoort HC, et al. Endoscopic or surgical step-up approach for infected necrotising pancreatitis: a multicentre randomised trial. Lancet 2018;391: 51-58.

[22] Bang JY, Arnoletti JY, Holt JP, et al. An endoscopic transluminal approach, compared to minimally invasive surgery, reduces complications and costs for patients with necrotizing pancreatitis. Gastroenterology 2019; 156: 1027-40.

[23] Nemoto Y, Attam R, Arain MA, et al. Interventions for walled off necrosis using an algorithm based endoscopic step-up approach: outcomes in a large cohort of patients. Pancreatology 2017;17: 663-68.

[24] Ross AS, Irani S, Gan SI, et al. Dual-modality drainage of infected and symptomatic walled-off pancreatic necrosis: long-term clinical outcomes. Gastrointest Endosc 2014; 79: 929-35.

[25] Ross A, Gluck M, Irani S, et al. Combined endoscopic and percutaneous drainage of organized pancreatic necrosis. Gastrointest Endosc 2010; 71: 79-84.

[26] Gluck M, Ross A, Irani S, et al. Dual modality drainage for symptomatic walled-off pancreatic necrosis reduces length of hospitalization, radiological procedures, and number of endoscopies compared to standard percutaneous drainage. J Gastrointest Surg 2012; 16: 248-57.

[27] Sahar N, Kozarek R, Kanji ZS, et al. Do lumen-apposing metal stents (LAMS) improve treatment outcomes of walled-off pancreatic necrosis over plastic stents using dual-modality drainage? Endosc Int Open 2017; 5: E1052-59.

[28] Bang JY, Navaneethan U, Hasan MK, Sutton B, Hawes R, Varadarajulu S. Non-superiority of lumen-apposing metal stents over plastic stents for drainage of walled-off necrosis in a randomised trial. Gut 2019; 68: 1200-09.

[29] Arvanitakis M, Dumonceau J-M, Albert J, et al. Endoscopic management of acute necrotizing pancreatitis: European Society of Gastrointestinal Endoscopy (ESGE) evidence-based multidisciplinary guidelines. Endoscopy 2018; 50: 524-46.

[30] Freeny PC, Hauptmann E, Althaus SJ, et al. Percuta- neous CT-guided catheter drainage of infected acute necrotizing pancreatitis: techniques and results. AJR Am J Roentgenol 1998;170:969-975.

[31] Horvath K, Freeny P, Escallon J, et al. Safety and efficacy of video-assisted retroperitoneal debridement for infected pancreatic collections: a multicenter, prospective, single-arm phase 2 study. Arch Surg 2010;145:817-825

[32] Todd H. Baron,Christopher J. DiMaio, Andrew Y. Wang, and Katherine A. Morgan. American Gastroenterological Association Clinical Practice Update: Management of Pancreatic Necrosis. Gastroenterology 2020;158:67-75.

[33] Munene G, Dixon E, Sutherland F. Open transgastric debridement and internal drainage of symptomatic non-infected walled-off pancreatic necrosis. HPB (Oxford) 2011;13:234-239.

[34] Gibson SC, Robertson BF, Dickson EJ, et al. 'Step-port' laparoscopic cystgastrostomy for the management of organized solid predominant post-acute fluid collections after severe acute pancreatitis. HPB (Oxford) 2014; 16:170-176.

[35] Worhunsky DJ, Qadan M, Dua MM, et al. Laparoscopic transgastric necrosectomy for the management of pancreatic necrosis. J Am Coll Surg 2014;219:735-743.

[36] Parikh PY, Pitt HA, Kilbane M, et al. Pancreatic necrosectomy: North American mortality is much lower than expected. J Am Coll Surg 2009;209:712-719.

[37] Rodriguez JR, Razo AO, Targarona J, et al. Debridement and closed packing for sterile or infected necrotizing pancreatitis: insights into indications and outcomes in 167 patients. Ann Surg 2008;247:294-299.

Section 2

Progress in Treatment of Pancreatitis

Chapter 3

Surgical and Interventional Management of Complications Caused by Pancreatitis

Tommaso Stecca, Bruno Pauletti, Luca Bonariol, Ezio Caratozzolo, Enrico Battistella, Silvia Zilio and Marco Massani

Abstract

Acute pancreatitis has a broad clinical spectrum: from mild, self-limited disease to fulminant illness resulting in multi-organ failure leading to a prolonged clinical course with up to 30% mortality in case of infected necrosis. Management of local complications such as pseudocysts and walled-off necrosis may vary from clinical observation to interventional treatment procedures. Gram negative bacteria infection may develop in up to one-third of patients with pancreatic necrosis leading to a clinical deterioration with the onset of the systemic inflammatory response syndrome and organ failure. When feasible, an interventional treatment is indicated. Percutaneous or endoscopic drainage approach are the first choices. A combination of minimally invasive techniques (step-up approach) is possible in patients with large or multiple collections. Open surgical treatment has been revised both in the timing and in the operating modalities in the last decades. Since 1990s, the surgical treatment of infected necrosis shifted to a more conservative approach. Disruption of the main pancreatic duct is present in up to 50% of patients with pancreatic fluid collections. According to the location along the Wirsung, treatment may vary from percutaneous drainage, endoscopic retrograde pancreatography with sphincterectomy or stenting to traditional surgical procedures. Patients may suffer from vascular complications in up to 23% of cases. Tissue disruption provoked by lipolytic and proteolytic enzymes, iatrogenic complications during operative procedures, splenic vein thrombosis, and pseudoaneurysms are the pathophysiological determinants of bleeding. Interventional radiology is the first line treatment and when it fails or is not possible, an urgent surgical approach should be adopted. Chylous ascites, biliary strictures and duodenal stenosis are complications that, although uncommon and transient, may have different treatment modalities from non-operative, endoscopic to open surgery.

Keywords: pancreatic pseudocysts, walled-off necrosis, infected pancreatic necrosis, disconnected pancreatic duct syndrome, vascular complications, chylous ascites

1. Introduction

The majority of patients suffering from acute pancreatitis will have a mild, self-limited and uncomplicated course. Pancreatic necrosis may develop in up to

10%-20% of patients, because of insufficient perfusion of pancreatic parenchyma to support metabolic requirements, leading to a prolonged clinical course with up to 30% mortality in case of infected necrosis [1]. Local and systemic complications, mild or life-threatening, such as pancreatic and/or peripancreatic fluid collections, walled-off necrosis, infected pancreatic necrosis, disconnected pancreatic duct syndrome and vascular complications can occur. The successful management of these patients needs a multidisciplinary team composed by gastroenterologists, surgeons, interventional radiologists, and specialists in critical care medicine, infectious disease, and nutrition. Intervention is generally required for infected pancreatic necrosis and less commonly in patients with sterile necrosis who are symptomatic (gastric or duodenal outlet or biliary obstruction) [2]. The surgical odyssey in managing necrotizing pancreatitis is a notable example of how evidence-based knowledge leads to improvement in patient care. Open surgical necrosectomy has been the traditional surgical treatment for years. However, although it provides a wide access but it is associated with high morbidity (34%-95%) and mortality (11-39%). In the last decades treatment has moved towards minimally invasive techniques: laparoscopy, retroperitoneal and endoscopic or percutaneous approaches. These can allow open surgery to be postponed in a sub-acute setting or even to avoid it [3–6].

2. Pancreatic necrosis and pseudocysts

Local complications such as pancreatic and/or peripancreatic fluid collections can occur after an episode of acute pancreatitis or after recrudescence of chronic pancreatitis or a blunt, penetrating, iatrogenic pancreatic trauma. Peripancreatic fluid collections, with or without a necrotic component, are early manifestations of the pancreatic inflammatory process. They are not delimited by a well-defined inflammatory wall and often remain asymptomatic, ending in spontaneous resolution by a gradual reduction in size. After four weeks from the clinical manifestation, persistent collections usually become wall-defined, encapsulated, with (walled-off necrosis) or without (pancreatic pseudocyst) a necrotic component and a varying degree of pancreatic parenchyma involvement [7].

Management of pseudocysts and walled-off pancreatic necrosis (WOPN) rely on patient's symptoms, location and characteristics of pancreatic and/or peripancreatic collections, local complications (such as pseudoaneurysm), expertise and availability of a multidisciplinary group [8].

In asymptomatic patients, clinical observation and periodic imaging follow up (every three-six months) represent the most successful management, due to the frequent reduction in size and spontaneous resolution of non-complicated homogeneous collections and to the morbidity associated to interventional (endoscopic or radiologic) treatment procedures. In these cases, it is possible to associate nutritional and pharmacological support (nasoenteric feeding reduces pain and improves nutritional status; proton pump inhibitors and somatostatin-analogue such as octreotide reduce pancreatic secretion).

Infection will develop in about one third of patients with pancreatic necrosis. It may arise at any time during the clinical course but peak incidence is between the 2nd and the 4th week after presentation [2]. Gram-negative bacteria are the main infectious species isolated, the most common of which are *Escherichia coli* and *Pseudomonas aeruginosa* [9]. Recently, a trend towards increasing incidence of Gram-positive and multi-resistant bacteria has been demonstrated [10, 11].

Prognosis and management are greatly affected by the recognition between sterile and infected pancreatic necrosis. Clues of suspicion should arise in case of clinical signs of systemic inflammatory response syndrome (SIRS) (new-onset fever, tachycardia, leukocytosis) or organ failure [12]. A blood culture with positive bacterial results and gas in and around the pancreas on a CT scan may give indirect evidence of infection. Prophylactic antibiotic use in patients suffering from acute pancreatitis has not been proven to decrease infection rate and thus, according to the meta-analysis by Wittau et al. [13] it is not recommended a routine prophylaxis. The Cochrane review by Villatoro et al. [14] showed that antibiotic prophylaxis was not associated with a reduced incidence of pancreatic necrosis infection, even though it was associated with significantly decreased mortality. CT- or US-guided fine needle aspiration of pancreatic necrosis for bacteriologic analysis are an accurate, safe and reliable techniques with high accuracy (89.4%-100%) [15, 16].

In symptomatic patients, with rapidly enlarging pseudocysts or systemic manifestations of organ failure sustained by an infectious process, an interventional treatment is indicated. In this case endoscopic drainage approach is the first choice, especially when fluid collection is close to gastroduodenal lumen. A combination of techniques is possible in patients with large collections, extended in pelvis and paracolic gutters, or multiple collections [17].

2.1 Endoscopic drainage

Endoscopic drainage of a walled collection is the preferred method when the drainage criteria are met: mature collections delimited by a well-defined inflammatory capsule and with a mostly liquid content; cystic wall adherent to stomach or duodenum; and collection's size at least 6 cm in size.

This procedure has to be performed by an endoscopist with expertise and when surgical or interventional radiology staffs are available [18]. Contraindications to endoscopic drainage are: presence of pseudoaneurysm due to gastroduodenal or splenic artery erosion, with high risk of bleeding; and collections without a mature wall.

Drainage techniques consist in [19]: *transmural drainage*: creation of a passage through the stomach or duodenum wall into the cyst lumen. This permits cystic drainage after balloon dilatation and placement of one or more stents. This method is preferred to drain WOPN in order to evacuate solid debris. T*ranspapillary drainage*: placement of a ductal pancreatic stent with or without preliminary sphincterotomy to drain cysts in communication with pancreatic duct, especially when endoscopic retrograde pancreatography demonstrates ongoing ductal leak.

Transmural approach is adopted when large and symptomatic walled-off pancreatic fluid collection is close to gastroduodenal structures. Transmural puncture through gastroduodenal wall (where is endoscopically visible a bulge resulting by apposition to the cyst), is nowadays ecoendoscopically guided. This permits to accurately identify puncture site for cystenterostomy, avoiding vessels or other interposed structures and evaluating real distance to pass through [20]. Self-expanding metal stents or plastic double pig-tail stents can be both used. Lumen Apposing Metal Stent (LAMS) are associated with higher bleeding grade but allow immediate procedures such as endoscopic necrosectomy.

Drainage of turbid necrotic fluid suggests debris presence and can be managed with direct endoscopic debridement and/or with the placement of a naso-cystic catheter for post-procedural lavage. Repeated debridement or association with percutaneous drainage or percutaneous endoscopic gastrostomy can be necessary with unresolved fluid collections [21].

For patients with small pseudocysts derived from main pancreatic duct, transpapillary stent placement is indicated as first drainage approach. This provides continuous drainage of pancreatic fluid, leading to resolution of pancreatic ductal disruption that is responsible of pseudocyst. Follow up with CT or EUS is preferred after four to six weeks if necrotic debridement was not necessary and stents are then removed the fluid cavity is collapsed. More frequent imaging is obtained in patients who underwent necrosectomy, to determine if additional debridement is necessary. When collections are completely evacuated, stents are removed. Long-term stents seem to protect against recurrence allowing ongoing drainage of pancreatic secretions, although cystenterostomy tract matures and persists after eventual stent removal [22].

2.2 Percutaneous drainage

Percutaneous drainage remains an important treatment modality for patients with symptomatic collections. It may be used both as primary therapy or as an adjunct to other techniques. According to the last International [23], American [1] and Japanese [24] guidelines, percutaneous catheter (or endoscopic transmural drainage) should be the first step in the treatment of patients with suspected or confirmed (walled-off) infected necrotizing pancreatitis. This is applied to decompress retroperitoneal fluid collections, to provide a rapid and effective means for source control in patients with infected pancreatic necrosis. It favors clinical stabilization of patients before endoscopic or surgical debridement and is the first choice when endoscopic drainage is unavailable, unsuccessful, or not technically feasible [25].

The positioning can be performed via the transperitoneal or retroperitoneal approaches. It is technically feasible in >95% of patients [26]. Retroperitoneal route is generally preferred because it avoids peritoneal contamination, enteric fistulas and facilitates a possible step-up approach (see "Surgical approach" chapter). Moreover, the catheter tract can act as an entry portal for minimally invasive debridement methods, such as video assisted retroperitoneal or endoscopic debridement [1]. Catheters range from 8 Fr to 30 Fr in diameter; they allow for bedside irrigation and clearance of necrotic material, can be manipulated and replaced according to the evolution of the collections [27].

Percutaneous drainage alone may provide definitive therapy for a subset of patients. The prospective observational multicenter study by Horvath K. et al. in 2010, found that the decrease in the size of the collection of at least 75% after the first 10-14 days predicts successful percutaneous treatment. In 2011, a large prospective multicenter study of treatment outcomes among patients with necrotizing pancreatitis demonstrated that catheter drainage was the first intervention in 63% of cases and did not require additional necrosectomy in 35% of patients [28]. Two prospective randomized trials from the Dutch Pancreatitis Study Group compared various approaches to the management of symptomatic WON. They demonstrated that percutaneous drainage alone was successful in 35%-51% of patients and that a minimally invasive step-up approach was related to a lower rate of pancreatic fistulas, length of hospital stay and death, as compared with open necrosectomy [26, 29].

The risk of pancreatocutaneous fistula formation is the major potential drawback of this technique. The multicentre randomised trial by van Brunschot S. et al. demonstrated that the rate of pancreatic fistula formation was significantly higher in the percutaneous (32%) as compared to the video-assisted retroperitoneal debridement (VARD) group (5%) [29]. The rate is as high as 45% in those with disconnected duct syndrome [30].

2.3 Surgical approach

The surgical odyssey in managing necrotizing pancreatitis is a notable example of how evidence-based knowledge leads to improvement in patient care. In the beginning of the 20th century surgeons such as Mayo Robson, Mickulicz, and Moynihan, in the context of the progression of anesthesia, were induced to deploy laparotomy in an effort to treat complications of severe acute pancreatitis [31]. Over the next decades surgical intervention became the therapy of choice despite a mortality rate greater than 50%. Extensive pancreatic resection became the treatment of choice in the 1960s and 1970s. Innovations and increased accuracy in radiological techniques led to new approaches for management. Surgeons were divided between those who reserved the intervention for cases of infected necrosis by proposing delayed exploration, and those who proposed early debridement for all patients with necrotizing pancreatitis. Since 1990s several studies proved that nonoperative management of patients with sterile pancreatic necrosis was superior to surgical intervention, and that delayed intervention provided improved surgical mortality rates. The treatment of infected necrosis shifted to a more conservative approach also thanks to a comprehensive knowledge of the physio-pathological process of the systemic inflammatory response and the adoption of novel antibiotics in curbing systemic toxicity and protecting against organ failure. Recently, endoscopic debridement and minimally invasive techniques has been introduced [31, 32].

The last guidelines of the Working Group of the International Association of Pancreatology (IAP)/American Pancreatic Association (APA) published in 2013 [23] and of the American Gastroenterological Association (AGA) published in 2020 [1] on the management of acute pancreatitis and pancreatic necrosis list the common indications for intervention. A symptomatic sterile pancreatic necrosis is an indication for intervention (either radiological, endoscopical or surgical). Symptoms can be represented by: gastric, intestinal, or biliary obstruction due to the mass effect of walled-off necrosis, pain, persistent unwellness in patients without signs of infection [1]. In case of infected pancreatic necrosis invasive procedures (e.g. percutaneous catheter drainage, endoscopic transluminal drainage/necrosectomy, minimally invasive or open necrosectomy) should be delayed, where possible, until at least 4 weeks after initial presentation to permit the collection to become "walled-off". A randomized clinical trial [33] that compared early surgery (within 72 h) and delayed surgery (11 days after onset) demonstrated mortality rates of 56% and 27%, respectively.

Percutaneous drainage, alone or in combination with other minimally invasive approaches, can be an effective means for source control in patients with infected pancreatic necrosis. A significant number of patients (23%–47%) will resolve their necrosis with percutaneous drainage alone. In those with persistent disease, a step up to operative intervention may be undertaken. The tract of the drain is utilized to access the retroperitoneal space for an intracavitary videoscopic necrosectomy by which drains are left in the cavity for lavage and fistula control [26, 34, 35]. The PANTER Study in 2010, a prospective randomized multicenter trial, compared the step-up approach to open necrosectomy and found a higher rate of new-onset multiple-organ failure in the open necrosectomy group (40% vs. 12%) and an equivalent mortality between the groups [26]. Surgical transgastric debridement is similar to endoscopic transgastric debridement, can be done laparoscopically or open, and is performed by an anterior gastrotomy to access the posterior wall of the stomach for transmural access to the necrosis cavity. Open surgical debridement is still an important resource in the management of these patients for the debridement of necrotic tissue.

Before surgical approach, abdominal imaging is helpful to determine intra-abdominal status. Diagnosis of infected pancreatic necrosis is made by identification of air bubbles in retroperitoneal necrosis (areas with lack of contrast enhancement) on CT scan. Diagnosis can be confirmed by CT-guided fine needle aspiration of necrotic material for culture. CT is also indicated to define extent and location of necrotic areas, for example into the mesenteric root and down the paracolic gutters; to demonstrate the presence of a disconnected pancreatic segment (a viable pancreatic portion separated by the rest of pancreas by a necrotic segment, that require external drainage to create a controlled external pancreatic fistula); and to evaluate the presence of other local complications, such as gastric outlet obstruction, splenic or portal vein thrombosis and colonic necrosis. Open debridement with external drainage still plays an important, albeit limited, role. After access to retroperitoneum, fluid is evacuated and necrotic dissection and debridement is made. In biliary pancreatitis, cholecystectomy should be practiced but it is associated with increased incidence of postoperative bile leak or biliary injury. Colon resection and colostomy have to be considered if mesocolon is involved in peripancreatic necrosis. A feeding enteral tube and at least two-four drainage tubes should be placed [36].

Video-assisted retroperitoneal debridement approach requires preoperative percutaneous retroperitoneal access. Radiological catheter insertion is a route to guide the subsequent procedure directly down into necrotic cavity and postoperative lavage. The advantage is minimizing the risk of peritoneal contamination, but the access is limited and precludes other procedures over debridement [34]. Postoperative complications are: intra-abdominal residual fluid collections, derived from pancreatic leak not well controlled by drains; bleeding, due to vascular lesion during debridement maneuvers or rupture of pseudoaneurysm, related to vascular erosion caused by mechanical drain damage or infection associated with uncontrolled pancreatic fistula; pancreatic fistulas: amylase-rich (concentration greater than three times the upper limit of normal serum amylase) fluid coming from drains; biliary injury; and pancreatic endocrine and exocrine insufficiency, that may requires supplemental insulin and oral pancreatic enzyme replacement.

Each approach has distinct peculiarities with pros and cons that must be weighted in each case planning: pattern of disease, physiology of the patient, expertise of the multidisciplinary team, and the resources of the center [1].

3. Disconnected pancreatic duct syndrome

The term disconnected pancreatic duct syndrome (DPDS) refers to a subset of patients suffering from a disruption of the main pancreatic duct leading to a normal upstream pancreatic gland having no communication with the gastrointestinal tract [1, 37]. Up to 50% of patients with pancreatic fluid collections might have an underlying disconnected duct. It is best recognized using secretin-stimulated magnetic resonance cholangiopancreatography [38]. DPDS can be the result of acute necrotizing pancreatitis, chronic pancreatitis, and pancreatic trauma. Pancreatic juice is still secreted from the disconnected gland resulting in different resolutions that are a continuum of the same pathophysiologic process: recurrent acute pancreatitis, internal persistent pancreatic fistula (most often presenting as a peripancreatic fluid collection), external fistula, pancreatic pleural effusion, pancreatic ascites, or disconnected pancreatic tail syndrome [39, 40].

Internal fistulae are the result of ductal disruptions that are not contained by the inflammatory response. Anterior ductal disruptions result in pancreatic ascites, posterior ones result in pancreatic pleural effusions. Positive testing for a collection rich in pancreatic enzyme gives the secure diagnosis. A percutaneous drainage is the initial treatment to obtain a controlled fistula that in 70-82% of cases results in a spontaneous closure.

External fistulae may develop after pseudocyst percutaneous drainage. The stricture or the obstruction of the Wirsung result in ductal hypertension thus increasing the chance of developing this complication. Endoscopic retrograde pancreatography (ERP) with sphincterotomy or transpapillary stenting should be then performed, both in internal and in external fistulae, to reduce resistance of pancreatic juice flow to the duodenum [41].

If the disruption is in the body or the tail (disconnected pancreatic tail syndrome), open distal pancreatectomy and debridement associated with drainage are the traditional surgical procedures. These are characterized by a high periprocedural morbidity that is counterweighted by the single procedure and a concise overall course. Distal pancreatectomy can be undertaken during the first 30–60 days of illness, in the subacute setting [1].

The high morbidity and mortality associated with open surgical procedures, especially for poor surgical candidates, recommend a minimally invasive endoscopic [42]. Partial duct disruption can be treated with endoscopic transpapillary stent bridging with a fistula resolution rate of 56%, according to Varadarajulu et al. [43]. One possible endoscopic approach in case of complete duct disruption is the use of permanent indwelling transmural stents that allow the creation and maintenance of a fistulous tract into the gastrointestinal lumen [42].

Correct choice of procedure, as well as correct choice of timing of intervention, are mandatory for success.

4. Vascular complications (haemorrhage, pseudoaneurysm and thrombosis)

Haemorrhage, pseudoaneurysm and thrombosis are the main vascular complications with an incidence ranging from 1% to 23% in patients with acute pancreatitis. Arterial complications are less frequent than venous complications (1.3-10% vs. 22%) [44].

The etiopathology of bleeding in patients with severe pancreatitis can be summarized in four main causes. The first one is due to the local spreading of lipolytic and proteolytic enzymes during a severe pancreatitis or necrosis that leads to the disruption of the tissue and the release of pancreatic fluids thus resulting in the arterial wall damage [45]. The second cause is related to a iatrogenic damage: improper surgical management of acute pancreatitis with an early operation for non-infected necrosis has been reported in Literature as a possible cause of wall arterial weakening thus leading to bleeding due to the activated enzymes [46]. Another iatrogenic source of damage is associated to the radiological positioning of drains that could give a direct trauma to the vessels and a continuous local inflammation that can diminish arterial wall integrity [47]. A third pathogenic mechanism is splenic vein thrombosis due to the necrotizing process, pseudocyst and severe inflammation that could lead to portal hypertension and, as a late sequelae, to esophageal varices formation [45]. The last remarkable pathogenic mechanism is the formation of a pseudoaneurysm that derived from the rupture of a vessels into a long-standing pseudocyst [48]. Symptoms are gastrointestinal bleeding, abdominal pain and splenomegaly and they depend on the localization of pseudoaneurysm. The most common vessels are splenic (35-50%), gastroduodenal (20%), and pancreaticoduodenal (20%) artery. Other vessels involved are tributaries of the gastric, colic and hepatic bloodstream [40, 49].

Ultrasound (US) and Computed Tomography (CT) are the gold standard to diagnose a vascular complication. Specially, CT imaging showed a higher sensibility in the diagnosis of pseudo-aneurysm, and US has an important role in identifying thrombosis or in patients with iodine allergy or renal insufficiency [50]. Enhanced-contrast CT locates necrotic areas, abscess cavity, pseudocysts, and bleeding site.

Angiography is the gold standard technique for the location and the control of the bleeding [45]. Interventional radiology is the first line treatment in both elective and emergency management of vascular complications. Angiography followed by trans-arterial embolization (TAE) is the gold standard management [51]. Different techniques can be used: the one preferred is the sandwich technique with coil located proximally and distally to the pseudoaneurysm to minimize the risk of potential rebleeding [52]. Haemostasis can be implemented with glue, N-butyl cyanoacrylate (NBCA), thrombin, ethiodised oil or gelfoam. Patients with unsuccessful TAE or in which is technically impossible, an emergency haemostatic surgery should be performed. Ligation of bleeding arteries is the technique of choice although related to a high rate of rebleeding. In extreme cases, open packing or salvage emergency pancreatectomy may represent the only chances for survival [45].

Vascular complications are rare but potentially fatal with a difficult management that is why they should be treated in a tertiary centre.

5. Chylous ascites

Pancreatitis is a rare cause of chylous ascites (CA) and in Literature, only few cases about acute pancreatitis are reported since its discovered in 1984 [53, 54]. Other causes related to CA are abdominal trauma, malignancies, sarcoidosis, lymphangiomatosis, yellow nail syndrome, cirrhosis, and mycobacterial infections [55]. CA diagnosis is based on the presence of a milky triglyceride- rich fluid collection in the peritoneal cavity. Patients complain about abdominal pain, distension, weight loss, oedema, anorexia, and weakness.

Diagnosis requires peritoneal fluid sampling with documentation of a lipid rich fluid, triglyceride concentration > 1.2 mM (110 mg/dl), peritoneal-to-plasma protein concentration ratio of >0.5 and presence of microscopic fat. The minimum daily volume of CA considered significant ranges between 100 ml to 600 ml [56, 57].

The pathogenesis is not completely clarified especially when CA is due to acute pancreatitis. The main possible reason is the spreading of proteolytic and lipolytic enzymes associated to necrosis of pancreatic tissue that damage the lymphatic vessels thus provoking a lymph leakage. Other possible reasons are AP related and include: splenic vein thrombosis leading to portal vein hypertension thus causing the rupture of lymphatic vessels; and the severe inflammation that could cause lymphatic vessels obstruction and lymphatic exudation [58, 59].

CA treatment is multimodal. Conservative treatment is based on total parenteral nutrition (TPN) or medium chain triglyceride (MCT)-high protein enteral feeding with or without addition of octreotide and reaches the resolution in two to six weeks in 60-100% of cases [60, 61]. Interventional and surgical approaches should be reserved for cases in which conservative treatment has failed. A second line therapy is bipedal lymphangiography (BPLAG) with lipiodol. This technique permits to identify the normal lymphatic stream and locate the leakage site or the obstruction site. The accumulation of injected lipiodol determines an inflammatory response that acts as an embolic agent and determines leakage resolution in up to 70% of cases [62].

Van der Gaag and colleagues has considered any duration of chylous ascites, longer than 14 days despite therapy, a requirement for surgical intervention [63]. Surgical treatment may vary from a peritoneovenous shunt to open surgical ligation of the leaking lymphatics [64]. Surgical approach should be chosen only in case of persistent CA despite treatment, symptomatic patients, or impossibility to perform interventional radiology.

6. Biliary and duodenal complications

Biliary stricture (BS) and duodenal stenosis (DS) are uncommon complication of AP. Pathogenesis of these events is strictly related to the anatomical position between the pancreatic head, the common bile duct and the duodenum. BS and DS are, in most cases, early and transient conditions associated to severe inflammation [65]. The main causes for temporary BS are inflammatory oedema and pseudocyst formation and enlargement in the area proximal to the pancreatic head that create a compression of the common bile duct, thus causing jaundice, nausea, vomit, abdominal pain, pruritus, and fatigue to the patient [66].

A duodenal early complication is gastric outlet obstruction related to the abnormal peristaltic wave and following ileus caused by the severe inflammation and the possible compression of the duodenal loop by the enlarged neck of the pancreas that cause a lumen obstruction [67].

BS ad DS usually solve with a conservative treatment intended to overcome the acute inflammatory phase. Pseudocyst management is resumed in previous chapters.

In many studies, late BS is associated to pancreatic duct disruption (PDD) with pancreatic juice leakage when duct of the head/neck of pancreas is involved in pancreatic necrosis [68]. When PDD is suspected, contrast-enhanced CT should be performed to confirm it and after that an endoscopic retrograde cholangiopancreatography (ERCP) to localize the leakage and positioning a stent [69]. If this procedure failed, and a progression of the common duct stricture has developed, surgical procedure is indicated [53].

The process that leads a transient DS to an irreversible one is still unclear. Literature suggests that the underlaying cause is a possible ischemic and thrombotic event. Indeed, inflammation may induce arterial narrowing and/or thrombosis of the pancreaticoduodenal circulation producing local ischemia and resulting in chronic fibrosis [70]. Patients who present intermittent symptomatic episodes of upper gastrointestinal tract obstruction should undergo surgical bypass, chosen considering the pathophysiology (gastrojejunostomy or gastroenterostomy with vagotomy to prevent marginal ulcer) [71].

7. Conclusion

The majority of patients suffering from acute pancreatitis will have a mild, self-limited and uncomplicated course. Local and systemic complications, mild or life-threatening, such as pancreatic and/or peripancreatic fluid collections, walled-off necrosis, infected pancreatic necrosis, disconnected pancreatic duct syndrome and vascular complications can occur.

The successful management of these patients needs a multidisciplinary team composed by gastroenterologists, surgeons, interventional radiologists, and specialists in critical care medicine, infectious disease, and nutrition. However, it must be considered that the requisite technical expertise and judgment for many of these procedures is not widely available in all centres. Intervention is generally required for infected pancreatic necrosis and less commonly in patients with sterile necrosis who are symptomatic. The surgical odyssey in managing necrotizing pancreatitis has been described. Operative approaches to the treatment of acute pancreatitis complications have undergone a dramatic transformation over the past few decades. Prospective, randomized trials have further clarified the value of the latest minimally invasive approaches to the treatment of this disease. This is the notable example of how evidence-based knowledge leads to improvement in patient care.

Conflict of interest

The authors declare no conflict of interest.

Author details

Tommaso Stecca*, Bruno Pauletti, Luca Bonariol, Ezio Caratozzolo,
Enrico Battistella, Silvia Zilio and Marco Massani
Surgery Department, First Surgical Unit, Treviso Regional Hospital,
Azienda ULSS2 Marca Trevigiana, Italy

*Address all correspondence to: tommaso.stecca@aulss2.veneto.it

References

[1] Baron TH, DiMaio CJ, Wang AY, Morgan KA. American Gastroenterological Association Clinical Practice Update: Management of Pancreatic Necrosis. Gastroenterology. 2020; 158: 67-75.e1. DOI:10.1053/j.gastro.2019.07.064.

[2] Bugiantella W, Rondelli F, Boni M, Stella P, Polistena A, et al. Necrotizing pancreatitis: A review of the interventions. Int J Surg. 2016; 28: S163–S171. DOI:10.1016/j.ijsu.2015.12.038.

[3] Traverso LW, Kozarek RA. Pancreatic necrosectomy: Definitions and technique. J Gastrointest Surg. DOI:10.1016/j.gassur.2004.05.013. Epub ahead of print 2005. DOI: 10.1016/j.gassur.2004.05.013.

[4] Tan V, Charachon A, Lescot T, Chafaï N, Le Baleur Y, et al. Endoscopic transgastric versus surgical necrosectomy in infected pancreatic necrosis. Clin Res Hepatol Gastroenterol. DOI:10.1016/j.clinre.2014.06.016. Epub ahead of print 2014. DOI: 10.1016/j.clinre.2014.06.016.

[5] Freeman ML, Werner J, Van Santvoort HC, Baron TH, Besselink MG, et al. Interventions for necrotizing pancreatitis: Summary of a multidisciplinary consensus conference. Pancreas. DOI:10.1097/MPA.0b013e318269c660. Epub ahead of print 2012. DOI: 10.1097/MPA.0b013e318269c660.

[6] Raraty MGT, Halloran CM, Dodd S, Ghaneh P, Connor S, et al. Minimal access retroperitoneal pancreatic necrosectomy: Improvement in morbidity and mortality with a less invasive approach. Ann Surg. DOI:10.1097/SLA.0b013e3181d96c53. Epub ahead of print 2010. DOI: 10.1097/SLA.0b013e3181d96c53.

[7] Cui ML, Kim KH, Kim HG, Han J, Kim H, et al. Incidence, risk factors and clinical course of pancreatic fluid collections in acute pancreatitis. Dig Dis Sci. DOI:10.1007/s10620-013-2967-4. Epub ahead of print 2014. DOI: 10.1007/s10620-013-2967-4.

[8] Bradley EL, Howard TJ, Van Sonnenberg E, Fotoohi M. Intervention in necrotizing pancreatitis: An evidence-based review of surgical and percutaneous alternatives. J Gastrointest Surg. DOI:10.1007/s11605-007-0445-z. Epub ahead of print 2008. DOI: 10.1007/s11605-007-0445-z.

[9] Lu J Di, Cao F, Ding YX, Wu YD, Guo YL, et al. Timing, distribution, and microbiology of infectious complications after necrotizing pancreatitis. World J Gastroenterol. DOI:10.3748/wjg.v25.i34.5162. Epub ahead of print 2019. DOI: 10.3748/wjg.v25.i34.5162.

[10] Schmidt PN, Roug S, Hansen EF, Knudsen JD, Novovic S. Spectrum of microorganisms in infected walled-off pancreatic necrosis - Impact on organ failure and mortality. Pancreatology. DOI:10.1016/j.pan.2014.09.001. Epub ahead of print 2014. DOI: 10.1016/j.pan.2014.09.001.

[11] Lee HS, Lee SK, Park DH, Lee SS, Seo DW, et al. Emergence of multidrug resistant infection in patients with severe acute pancreatitis. Pancreatology. DOI:10.1016/j.pan.2014.10.003. Epub ahead of print 2014. DOI: 10.1016/j.pan.2014.10.003.

[12] Rau BM, Bothe A, Kron M, Beger HG. Role of Early Multisystem Organ Failure as Major Risk Factor for Pancreatic Infections and Death in Severe Acute Pancreatitis. Clin Gastroenterol Hepatol. DOI:10.1016/j.cgh.2006.05.030. Epub ahead of print 2006. DOI: 10.1016/j.cgh.2006.05.030.

[13] Wittau M, Mayer B, Scheele J, Henne-Bruns D, Dellinger EP, et al.

Systematic review and meta-analysis of antibiotic prophylaxis in severe acute pancreatitis. Scandinavian Journal of Gastroenterology. DOI:10.3109/00365521.2010.531486. Epub ahead of print 2011. DOI: 10.3109/00365521.2010.531486.

[14] Villatoro E, Mulla M, Larvin M. Antibiotic therapy for prophylaxis against infection of pancreatic necrosis in acute pancreatitis. Cochrane Database Syst Rev. DOI:10.1002/14651858.cd002941.pub3. Epub ahead of print 2010. DOI: 10.1002/14651858.cd002941.pub3.

[15] Banks PA, Gerzof SG, Langevin RE, Silverman SG, Sica GT, et al. CT-guided aspiration of suspected pancreatic infection - Bacteriology and clinical outcome. Int J Pancreatol. DOI:10.1007/BF02784951. Epub ahead of print 1995. DOI: 10.1007/BF02784951.

[16] Rau B, Pralle U, Mayer JM, Beger HG. Role of ultrasonographically guided fine-needle aspiration cytology in the diagnosis of infected pancreatic necrosis. Br J Surg. DOI:10.1046/j.1365-2168.1998.00707.x. Epub ahead of print 1998. DOI: 10.1046/j.1365-2168.1998.00707.x.

[17] Werner J, Feuerbach S, Uhl W, Büchler MW. Management of acute pancreatitis: From surgery to interventional intensive care. Gut. DOI:10.1136/gut.2003.035907. Epub ahead of print 2005. DOI: 10.1136/gut.2003.035907.

[18] Muthusamy VR, Chandrasekhara V, Acosta RD, Bruining DH, Chathadi K V., et al. The role of endoscopy in the diagnosis and treatment of inflammatory pancreatic fluid collections. Gastrointest Endosc. DOI:10.1016/j.gie.2015.11.027. Epub ahead of print 2016. DOI: 10.1016/j.gie.2015.11.027.

[19] Binmoeller KF, Seifert H, Walter A, Soehendra N. Transpapillary and transmural drainage of pancreatic pseudocysts. Gastrointest Endosc. DOI:10.1016/S0016-5107(95)70095-1. Epub ahead of print 1995. DOI: 10.1016/S0016-5107(95)70095-1.

[20] Park DH, Lee SS, Moon SH, Choi SY, Jung SW, et al. Endoscopic ultrasound-guided versus conventional transmural drainage for pancreatic pseudocysts: A prospective randomized trial. Endoscopy. DOI:10.1055/s-0029-1215133. Epub ahead of print 2009. DOI: 10.1055/s-0029-1215133.

[21] Seewald S, Groth S, Omar S, Imazu H, Seitz U, et al. Aggressive endoscopic therapy for pancreatic necrosis and pancreatic abscess: A new safe and effective treatment algorithm (videos). Gastrointest Endosc. DOI:10.1016/S0016-5107(05)00541-9. Epub ahead of print 2005. DOI: 10.1016/S0016-5107(05)00541-9.

[22] Weckman L, Kylänpää ML, Puolakkainen P, Halttunen J. Endoscopic treatment of pancreatic pseudocysts. Surg Endosc Other Interv Tech. DOI:10.1007/s00464-005-0201-y. Epub ahead of print 2006. DOI: 10.1007/s00464-005-0201-y.

[23] Iap WG, Acute APA, Guidelines P. IAP/APA evidence-based guidelines for the management of acute pancreatitis. Pancreatology. 2013; 13: 1-15. DOI:10.1016/j.pan.2013.07.063.

[24] Isaji S, Takada T, Kawarada Y, Hirata K, Mayumi T, et al. JPN Guidelines for the management of acute pancreatitis: Surgical management. J Hepatobiliary Pancreat Surg. 2006; 13: 48-55. DOI:10.1007/s00534-005-1051-7.

[25] Keane MG, Sze SF, Cieplik N, Murray S, Johnson GJ, et al. Endoscopic versus percutaneous drainage of symptomatic pancreatic fluid

collections: a 14-year experience from a tertiary hepatobiliary centre. Surg Endosc. DOI:10.1007/s00464-015-4668-x. Epub ahead of print 2016. DOI: 10.1007/s00464-015-4668-x.

[26] van Santvoort HC, Besselink MG, Bakker OJ, Hofker HS, Boermeester MA, et al. A Step-up Approach or Open Necrosectomy for Necrotizing Pancreatitis. N Engl J Med. DOI:10.1056/nejmoa0908821. Epub ahead of print 2010. DOI: 10.1056/nejmoa0908821.

[27] Mortelé KJ, Girshman J, Szejnfeld D, Ashley SW, Erturk SM, et al. CT-guided percutaneous catheter drainage of acute necrotizing pancreatitis: Clinical experience and observations in patients with sterile and infected necrosis. Am J Roentgenol. DOI:10.2214/AJR.08.1116. Epub ahead of print 2009. DOI: 10.2214/AJR.08.1116.

[28] Van Santvoort HC, Bakker OJ, Bollen TL, Besselink MG, Ahmed Ali U, et al. A conservative and minimally invasive approach to necrotizing pancreatitis improves outcome. Gastroenterology. DOI:10.1053/j.gastro.2011.06.073. Epub ahead of print 2011. DOI: 10.1053/j.gastro.2011.06.073.

[29] van Brunschot S, van Grinsven J, van Santvoort HC, Bakker OJ, Besselink MG, et al. Endoscopic or surgical step-up approach for infected necrotising pancreatitis: a multicentre randomised trial. Lancet. DOI:10.1016/S0140-6736(17)32404-2. Epub ahead of print 2018. DOI: 10.1016/S0140-6736(17)32404-2.

[30] Ross A, Gluck M, Irani S, Hauptmann E, Fotoohi M, et al. Combined endoscopic and percutaneous drainage of organized pancreatic necrosis. Gastrointest Endosc. DOI:10.1016/j.gie.2009.06.037. Epub ahead of print 2010. DOI: 10.1016/j.gie.2009.06.037.

[31] Bradley EL, Dexter ND. Management of severe acute pancreatitis: A surgical odyssey. Annals of Surgery. DOI:10.1097/SLA.0b013e3181c72b79. Epub ahead of print 2010. DOI: 10.1097/SLA.0b013e3181c72b79.

[32] Banks PA. Acute pancreatitis: Landmark studies, management decisions, and the future. Pancreas. 2016; 45: 633-640. DOI:10.1097/MPA.0000000000000632.

[33] Mier J, Luque-De León E, Castillo A, Robledo F, Blanco R. Early versus late necrosectomy in severe necrotizing pancreatitis. Am J Surg. DOI:10.1016/S0002-9610(96)00425-4. Epub ahead of print 1997. DOI: 10.1016/S0002-9610(96)00425-4.

[34] Horvath K, Freeny P, Escallon J, Heagerty P, Comstock B, et al. Safety and efficacy of video-assisted retroperitoneal debridement for infected pancreatic collections: A multicenter, prospective, single-arm phase 2 study. Arch Surg. DOI:10.1001/archsurg.2010.178. Epub ahead of print 2010. DOI: 10.1001/archsurg.2010.178.

[35] Freeny PC, Hauptmann E, Althaus SJ, Traverso LW, Sinanan M. Percutaneous CT-guided catheter drainage of infected acute necrotizing pancreatitis: Techniques and results. Am J Roentgenol. DOI:10.2214/ajr.170.4.9530046. Epub ahead of print 1998. DOI: 10.2214/ajr.170.4.9530046.

[36] Uhl W, Warshaw A, Imrie C, Bassi C, McKay CJ, et al. IAP Guidelines for the Surgical Management of Acute Pancreatitis. Pancreatology. DOI:10.1159/000071269. Epub ahead of print 2003. DOI: 10.1159/000071269.

[37] Kozarek RA, Ball TJ, Patterson DJ, Freeny PC, Ryan JA, et al. Endoscopic transpapillary therapy for disrupted pancreatic duct and peripancreatic fluid collections. Gastroenterology.

DOI:10.1016/0016-5085(91)90790-r. Epub ahead of print 1991. DOI: 10.1016/0016-5085(91)90790-r.

[38] Bang JY, Wilcox CM, Navaneethan U, Hasan MK, Peter S, et al. Impact of Disconnected Pancreatic Duct Syndrome on the Endoscopic Management of Pancreatic Fluid Collections. Ann Surg. DOI:10.1097/SLA.0000000000002082. Epub ahead of print 2018. DOI: 10.1097/SLA.0000000000002082.

[39] DiMaio CJ. Management of complications of acute pancreatitis. Curr Opin Gastroenterol. 2018; 34: 336-342. DOI:10.1097/MOG.0000000000000462.

[40] Martin RF, Hein AR. Operative Management of Acute Pancreatitis. Surgical Clinics of North America. DOI:10.1016/j.suc.2013.02.007. Epub ahead of print 2013. DOI: 10.1016/j.suc.2013.02.007.

[41] Morgan KA, Adams DB. Management of Internal and External Pancreatic Fistulas. Surgical Clinics of North America. DOI:10.1016/j.suc.2007.08.008. Epub ahead of print 2007. DOI: 10.1016/j.suc.2007.08.008.

[42] Nadkarni NA, Kotwal V, Sarr MG, Vege SS. Disconnected pancreatic duct syndrome endoscopic stent or surgeon's knife? Pancreas. DOI:10.1097/MPA.0000000000000216. Epub ahead of print 2015. DOI: 10.1097/MPA.0000000000000216.

[43] Varadarajulu S, Noone TC, Tutuian R, Hawes RH, Cotton PB. Predictors of outcome in pancreatic duct disruption managed by endoscopic transpapillary stent placement. Gastrointest Endosc. DOI:10.1016/S0016-5107(04)02832-9. Epub ahead of print 2005. DOI: 10.1016/S0016-5107(04)02832-9.

[44] Evans RPT, Mourad MM, Pall G, Fisher SG, Bramhall SR. Pancreatitis: Preventing catastrophic haemorrhage. World Journal of Gastroenterology. DOI:10.3748/wjg.v23.i30.5460. Epub ahead of print 2017. DOI: 10.3748/wjg.v23.i30.5460.

[45] Flati G, Andrén-Sandberg Å, La Pinta M, Porowska B, Carboni M. Potentially fatal bleeding in acute pancreatitis:Pathophysiology,prevention, and treatment. Pancreas. DOI:10.1097/00006676-200301000-00002. Epub ahead of print 2003. DOI: 10.1097/00006676-200301000-00002.

[46] Tsiotos GG, Juarez MM, Sarr MG. Intraabdominal hemorrhage complicating surgical management of necrotizing pancreatitis. Pancreas. DOI:10.1097/00006676-199603000-00003. Epub ahead of print 1996. DOI: 10.1097/00006676-199603000-00003.

[47] Beger HG, Büchler M, Bittner R, Block S, Nevalainen T, et al. Necrosectomy and postoperative local lavage in necrotizing pancreatitis. Br J Surg. DOI:10.1002/bjs.1800750306. Epub ahead of print 1988. DOI: 10.1002/bjs.1800750306.

[48] M.A. V, E. V, F. P, F. S, L. F, et al. Pseudoaneurysm of the gastroduodenal artery secondary to chronic pancreatitis. Annals of Vascular Surgery.

[49] Bergert H, Hinterseher I, Kersting S, Leonhardt J, Bloomenthal A, et al. Management and outcome of hemorrhage due to arterial pseudoaneurysms in pancreatitis. Surgery. DOI:10.1016/j.surg.2004.10.009. Epub ahead of print 2005. DOI: 10.1016/j.surg.2004.10.009.

[50] Chiang KC, Chen TH, Hsu J Te. Management of chronic pancreatitis complicated with a bleeding pseudoaneurysm. World J Gastroenterol. 2014; 20: 16132-16137. DOI:10.3748/wjg.v20.i43.16132.

[51] Zhang C, Li A, Luo T, Li J, Liu D, et al. Strategy and management of

severe hemorrhage complicating pancreatitis and post-pancreatectomy. Diagnostic Interv Radiol. DOI:10.5152/dir.2018.18283. Epub ahead of print 2019. DOI: 10.5152/dir.2018.18283.

[52] Kirby JM, Vora P, Midia M, Rawlinson J. Vascular complications of pancreatitis: Imaging and intervention. Cardiovasc Intervent Radiol. DOI:10.1007/s00270-007-9138-y. Epub ahead of print 2008. DOI: 10.1007/s00270-007-9138-y.

[53] Karakayali FY. Surgical and interventional management of complications caused by acute pancreatitis. World J Gastroenterol. 2014; 20: 13412-13423. DOI:10.3748/wjg.v20.i37.13412.

[54] Goldfarb JP. Chylous Effusions Secondary to Pancreatitis: Case Report and Review of the Literature. Am J Gastroenterol. DOI:10.1111/j.1572-0241.1984.tb05101.x. Epub ahead of print 1984. DOI: 10.1111/j.1572-0241.1984.tb05101.x.

[55] Steinemann DC, Dindo D, Clavien PA, Nocito A. Atraumatic chylous ascites: Systematic review on symptoms and causes. Journal of the American College of Surgeons. DOI:10.1016/j.jamcollsurg.2011.01.010. Epub ahead of print 2011. DOI: 10.1016/j.jamcollsurg.2011.01.010.

[56] Weniger M, D'Haese JG, Angele MK, Kleespies A, Werner J, et al. Treatment options for chylous ascites after major abdominal surgery: a systematic review. Am J Surg. DOI:10.1016/j.amjsurg.2015.04.012. Epub ahead of print 2016. DOI: 10.1016/j.amjsurg.2015.04.012.

[57] Cárdenas A, Chopra S. Chylous ascites. American Journal of Gastroenterology. DOI:10.1016/S0002-9270(02)04268-5. Epub ahead of print 2002. DOI: 10.1016/S0002-9270(02)04268-5.

[58] Al-Ghamdi MY, Bedi A, Reddy SB, Tanton RT, Peltekian KM. Chylous ascites secondary to pancreatitis: Management of an uncommon entity using parenteral nutrition and octreotide. Dig Dis Sci. DOI:10.1007/s10620-006-9734-8. Epub ahead of print 2007. DOI: 10.1007/s10620-006-9734-8.

[59] Poo S, Pencavel TD, Jackson J, Jiao LR. Portal hypertension and chylous ascites complicating acute pancreatitis: The therapeutic value of portal vein stenting. Ann R Coll Surg Engl. DOI:10.1308/rcsann.2017.0078. Epub ahead of print 2018. DOI: 10.1308/rcsann.2017.0078.

[60] Gómez-Martín JM, Martínez-Molina E, Sanjuanbenito A, Martín-Illana E, Arrieta F, et al. Chylous ascytes secondary to acute pancreatitis: a case report and review of literature. Nutr Hosp. DOI:10.1590/S0212-16112012000100044. Epub ahead of print 2012. DOI: 10.1590/S0212-16112012000100044.

[61] Gurusamy KS, Koti R, Fusai G, Davidson BR. Somatostatin analogues for pancreatic surgery. Cochrane Database of Systematic Reviews. DOI:10.1002/14651858.CD008370.pub3. Epub ahead of print 2013. DOI: 10.1002/14651858.CD008370.pub3.

[62] Tabchouri N, Frampas E, Marques F, Blanchard C, Jirka A, et al. Chylous Ascites Management After Pancreatic Surgery. World J Surg. DOI:10.1007/s00268-016-3772-y. Epub ahead of print 2017. DOI: 10.1007/s00268-016-3772-y.

[63] van der Gaag NA, Verhaar AC, Haverkort EB, Busch ORC, van Gulik TM, et al. Chylous Ascites after Pancreaticoduodenectomy: Introduction of a Grading System. J Am Coll Surg. DOI:10.1016/j.jamcollsurg.2008.07.007. Epub ahead of print 2008. DOI: 10.1016/j.jamcollsurg.2008.07.007.

[64] Assumpcao L, Cameron JL, Wolfgang CL, Edil B, Choti MA, et al. Incidence and management of chyle leaks following pancreatic resection: A high volume single-center institutional experience. J Gastrointest Surg. DOI:10.1007/s11605-008-0619-3. Epub ahead of print 2008. DOI: 10.1007/s11605-008-0619-3.

[65] Vijungco JD, Prinz RA. Management of Biliary and Duodenal Complications of Chronic Pancreatitis. World Journal of Surgery. DOI:10.1007/s00268-003-7246-7. Epub ahead of print 2003. DOI: 10.1007/s00268-003-7246-7.

[66] Creaghe SB, Roseman DM, Saik RP. Biliary obstruction in chronic pancreatitis: Indications for surgical intervention. Am Surg.

[67] BRUST RJ, CHEN KC. Acute hemorrhagic pancreatitis complicated by duodenalobstruction. Report of a case. Am J Roentgenol Radium Ther Nucl Med. 1962; 87: 732-735.

[68] Sugimoto M, Sonntag DP, Flint GS, Boyce CJ, Kirkham JC, et al. Biliary stenosis and gastric outlet obstruction: Late complications after acute pancreatitis with pancreatic duct disruption. Pancreas. DOI:10.1097/MPA.0000000000001064. Epub ahead of print 2018. DOI: 10.1097/MPA.0000000000001064.

[69] Bill JG, Mullady DK. Stenting for Benign and Malignant Biliary Strictures. Gastrointestinal Endoscopy Clinics of North America. DOI:10.1016/j.giec.2018.12.001. Epub ahead of print 2019. DOI: 10.1016/j.giec.2018.12.001.

[70] Archer S, Levitt S, Drury P. DUODENAL NECROSIS AND INTRAMURAL HAEMATOMA COMPLICATING ACUTE PANCREATITIS. Aust N Z J Surg. DOI:10.1111/j.1445-2197.1991.tb00286.x. Epub ahead of print 1991. DOI: 10.1111/j.1445-2197.1991.tb00286.x.

[71] Sharma H, Marwah S, Singla P, Garg A, Bhukkal B. Roux-en-Y duodenojejunostomy for surgical management of isolated duodenal obstruction due to chronic pancreatitis. Int J Surg Case Rep. DOI:10.1016/j.ijscr.2017.01.008. Epub ahead of print 2017. DOI: 10.1016/j.ijscr.2017.01.008.

Chapter 4

Endoscopic Retrograde Cholangiopancreatography in Acute Biliary Pancreatitis

Ülkü Saritaş and Yücel Üstündağ

Abstract

Acute pancreatitis (AP) is the most serious emergent disease in the gastroenterology field. The most common cause of AP is naturally gallstones. The most cases have mild disease and the illness limits itself in a short time period. In 15–20% of cases, the severe form of acute biliary pancreatitis (ABP) develops. Some patients have concomitant cholangitis. In these patients, releiving biliary obstruction with endoscopic retrograde cholangiography (ERCP) and endoscopic sphincterotomy (ES) is essential. However, correct timing of ERCP is a debate. While some authors and guidelines suggested that ERCP can be performed in first 24 hours, the others suggested its use during the first 72 hours. In the first 24 hours, ERCP is diffucult to apply due to ampullary edema and general ill situation of the patient. Rather than ERCP, agressive fluid replacement and supportive therapy are very much important in the first 72 hours of admission. Moreover, there is no consensus on timing of ERCP in patients with severe pancreatitis without cholangitis. But all international guidelines suggested that ERCP should be perfomed in all patients with mild or severe pancreatitis together with concomitant cholangitis during the first 72 hours. After resolution of ABP, cholecystectomy should be performed to prevent recurrent pancreatitis during the same hospitalization period (index cholecystectomy). If the patient is not suitable for cholecystectomy, ERCP and ES should be done to prevent further attacks of acute pancreatitis.

Keywords: acute biliary pancreatitis, urgent ERCP, early ERCP, endoscopic sphincterotomy, biliary duct stone

1. Introduction

Acute pancreatitis (AP) is the most serious emergent disease in the gastroenterology field. The most common cause of AP is naturally gallstones. The most cases have mild disease and the illness limits itself in a short time period. In 15–20% of cases, the severe form of AP develops. The triage of patients with AP in accordance with the severity of illness is the single most important factor affecting monitorisation and treatment protocol of these patients. Acute biliary pancreatitis (ABP) develops due to gall stones and or sludge mostly coming from gall bladder, impacted in ampulla Vateri (AV) leading to increased pancreatic ductal pressure, pancreatic edema, inflammation and possibly necrosis. A lot of human and animal studies displayed that biliary obstrucition lasting more than 48 hours creates pancreatic necrosis. Therefore, before the endoscopic retrograde cholangiography (ERCP) area, surgery was used to induce biliary decompression and impede progression into pancreatic necrosis, however, new quests started after facing high rate of morbidities and mortalities associated with surgery.

Introduction of ERCP and endoscopic sphincterotomy into the daily practice, endoscopic relieving of biliary obstruction has come into reality. Nevertheless, occurence of complications even mortalitiy in association with ERCP initiated new debate about its indications and timing in patients with ABP. Although for the last 30 years, there has been many ongoing studies about to whom and when ERCP will be performed in ABP, a certain conclusion has not been encountered yet. There has been 2 main strategies on debate [1].

1. Early routine ERCP strategy: If acute gallstone pancreatitis is triggered by duct obstruction caused by a stone, it would be reasonable to suggest that early ERCP with removal of any residual stones might reduce the severity of pancreatitis. The strategy of early ERCP is strongly supported by results from experimental studies and human studies, which show that the duration of biliary obstruction is a major factor in determining the severity of pancreatitis and that decompression of the biliary system can prevent progression of the disease. In addition, patients with severe pancreatitis tended to have stones impacted in the ampulla, and early (within 48 hours) surgical decompression of the obstruction has been shown to decrease mortalite rates These observations lend support to the theory of using early ERCP to remove obstructing stones in acute gallstone pancreatitis.

2. Early conservative management with or without delayed or selective use of ERCP strategy: Proponents of early conservative management with selective use of ERCP argue that early routine ERCP may lead to many unnecessary ERCPs in the majority of patients as the offending gallstone has often passed before the diagnosis of pancreatitis is made. Also, it remains unclear whether early ERCP improves the prognosis of acute gallstone pancreatitis. The severity of the pancreatitis may be determined at its inception and may not be dependent on the duration of duct obstruction. Furthermore, performing ERCP in the setting of acute pancreatitis can be technically difficult because of swollen ampulla and duodenal wall. Thus, it may be prudent to identify patients with persistent duct obstruction who would benefit from ERCP after a period of conservative medical management in order to avoid unnecessary negative ERCPs.

Due to 2 different approaches, how an imminent ERCP will affect the existing clinical situation in patients with ABP holds its uncertainity. There has been also no agreement on the preference of an urgent ERCP (U-ERCP) within 24 hours of patients'admission or an emergent ERCP (E-ERCP) within 48–72 hours [2]. These terms; U-ERCP and E-ERCP have been used in recent reports and the first paper published by Neoptolemos and et al. defined U-ERCP and E-ERCP differently than the other papers; the first one within 72 hours and the later within 35 days after admission [3]. Later on, ERCP within first 72 hours was labeled as U-ERCP [4] and after the year of 2000, U-ERCP has been defined as ERCP within 24 hours and E-ERCP as ERCP within 24–72 hours [2]. In severe ABP, there are some risks such as patient's bad general situation, technical difficulties due to pancreatic edema and potential interruption of aggressive fluid resuscitation during and after the ERCP procedure. Therefore, valid only for patients having persisting indication for biliary decompression, seveal authors and our clinical experience favor E-ERCP together with immense supportive treament of these patients rather than U-ERCP in the absence of life threatining cholangitis.

In severe cases with AP, there can be pain, fever, cholestasis, mental confusion and hypotension due to ongoing pancreatic inflammation and necrosis and under this circumstances, an imminent ERCP can make the situation even worser [5]. Although, if we scrutinize the real life data, we will see that there is some kind of pressure on ERCP physicians to perform ERCP at night and or at weekends by the physicians seeing these patients with ABP in the emergency room [6]. However, in severe ABP, it would be impossible to guarentee the co-existence of cholangitis only by looking at some clinical and biochemical parameters, the use of harmless non-invasive methods such as magnetic resonance cholangiography (MRCP) and or endoscopic ultrasonography (EUS) seems to be more reasonable. Hence, endoscopist who will perform ERCP should estimate the clinical situation of patient with ABP correctly and know very well to whom and when ERCP should be done. Thirty four years after the first report by Neoptolemus [3] suggesting wider application of ERCP with ES during AP, Schepers NJ [4] reported a multicentric article (APEC study) which underlined the fact that U-ERCP with ES does not reduce AP associated complications and mortality compated with conservative approaches. These authors supported a conservative strategy in severe ABP with ERCP indicated only in patients with cholangitis or persistant cholestasis.

In this chapter, we will mention about the role of ERCP during ABP in accordance with the clinical studies and meta-analysis published on this subject and we will add our self clinical experience and practice in this area. The order of titles will be as such,

- The pathogenesis and natural history of ABP
- The estimation of cholangitis and cholestasis
- The treatment steps in the first 72 hours in reference to International Guideliness
- To whom and when ERCP should be done during ABP?

2. The pathogenesis and natural history of ABP

In the setting of ABP, biliary stones or sludge material impacted in ampulla vateri induce transient obstruction in the biliary tree and pancreatic ductus, followed by reflux of bile into the pancreatic channel. Consequently, undraining pancreatic channel develops increased ductal pressure leading to backflow of activated pancreatic enzymes into the parenchyma. This starts a cascade of tissue injury with a spectrum of events starting with mild parencymal inflammation ending with loss of pancreatic parenchyma due to severe necrosis [7]. For sure, cholestasis and or cholangitis due to biliary obstruction in addititon to pancreatic inflammation can add into the clinical scenario. There are several evidences indicating the duration of obstruction correlates with te severity of pathology in the pancreas. These evidences reveal that persisting obstruction after 48 hours leads to different degrees of necrosis and if the ductal decompression is obtained before that time period, disease associated morbidity and mortality decreases significiantly [8–16]. Runzi et al. [8] used an animal model of AP by balloon obstructed biliopancreatic ductal system and they relieved the obstruction at 1th, 3rd and 5th days. The authors documented that the severity of parenchymal inflammation, fat necrosis, hemorrhage, acinar cell vacuolisaiton and necrosis were most prominent in animals with obstructed ductal sysytem at 5 th days of the experiment. On contrary, animals having decompressed ductal sysytem at 1th and 3 rd day of experiment, pancreatic injury was able to be avoided. Another report by Acosta et al. [11] investigating the same subject on a clinical study put forth that severe pancreatitis develops significantly more in patients with the obstruction lasting more than 48 hours compared to those having less than 48 hours of obstruction. These authors suggested to wait for 48 hours to implement an ERCP as the impacted stone may fall down spontaneously and if the signs of obstruction persists after 48 hours, then we should think about ERCP. On the grounds that at least half of the cases, the impacted stone in Ampulla Vateri will fall down spontaneously within 24–48 hours after ampullary and duodenal edema diminishes, we know that the pancreatitis in these patients will limit itself and recover within a few days. Acosta et al. [12] investigated the effects of early ductal decompression in a report and they compared 30 patients who underwent ERCP within first 48 hours with 31 patients who got only conservative treatment. Within the first group, 16 had passed the stone into the duodenum during 48 hours and only 14 patients underwent ERCP in whom 11 were shown to have impacted stones. In the second group of patients, 22 patients had got rid of obstuction spontaneously and 9 patients who had persistent signs of obstruction underwent ERCP and only 3 of them had impacted stone. As a result, %78 of patients passed stones spontaneously into the duodenum and E-ERCP was performed on the others within 48 hours without an uneventful clinical course and mortality. Another report by Cavdar et al. [13] indicated that 74% of patients with ABP passed stones into the duodenum within 72 hours of admission.

Based on all this data and our clinical experience about the natural progression of ABP, we suggest conservative approach during the first 24 to 48 hours to limitate the severity of pancreatitis by agressive fluid recessuation correction hypovolemia and organ hypoperfusion. This approach also allows us to evaluate the patients with regard to the presence of cholestasis and cholangitis and to find out which patients need ductal decompression.

APACHE II, Ranson, Glasgow veya Atlanta criteria are used to evaluate the severity of AP. Cholangitis and or cholestasis are assessed according to the presence or absence of severe pain, mental confusion, hipotansiyon, jaundice, elevated serum bilirubin ve liver enzymes and absence of bile in the aspirated gastric juice. Acosta and et al. [14] clearly demonstrated that absence of bile in the aspirated gastric juice hyperbilirubinemia and severe pain are the parameters most sensitive and spesific for the ongoing obstruction of AV. The authors concluded to apply ERCP to this subgroup of patients. However, these findings may also occur in patients with severe pancreatitis and do not indicate the existence of cholangitis. Thus, ERCP performed based only on these findings may worsen pancreatitis, even end up with death. Therefore, we need better methods to show the stone in the biliary tree. Before the area of MRCP and endoscopic ultrasonography (EUS), we would do diagnostic ERCP and endoscopic sphincterotomy in every patient with a diagnosis of ABP even if we did not detect gall stones in the bile duct. This policy has changed to 'never do diagnostic ERCP in ABP' and do first MRCP or if possible more sensitive EUS to decide if ERCP will be done or not.

3. The estimation of cholangitis and cholestasis

On clinical practice, the presence of cholangitis and or cholestasis in a patient with ABP is estimated by clinical and biochemical parameters together with abdominal ultrasonography (USG) [15–19]. Severe abdominal pain, fever, mental confusion, hypotension and jaundice can be seen in severe acute pancreatitis even in the absence of cholangitis. In 20% of patients, the liver enzymes can be persistently normal. The sensitivity of abdominal USG is very low around 27–50% in the diagnosis of cholestasis and cholangitis. The bile duct diameter can persist several days after spontaneously passing stones. Thus, we need more sensitive methods to detect cholangitis and or cholestasis. Nearly 20 years ago, ERCP has been widely used for a diagnostic purpose. However, there have been important developments with the administration of MRCP and EUS into the gastroenterology practice [20–29]. EUS is better than MRCP to detect gall stones smaller than 5 mm and after detecting the stone by EUS and as an adavantage of this procedure, ERCP can be used to extract the stone from the bile duct at the same session after EUS procedure [21–27]. Moon and his collagues [28] reported the accuracy rates of USG, computed tomography, MRCP, ERCP and intraductal USG to detect bile duct stones are 20%, 40%, %80%, 90%, 95%, respectively. The authors underlined IDUS and ERCP as the most sensitive methods to detect a CBD stone and suggested to use MRCP to choose the suitable patient for ERCP. They also notified that the rate of agreement between ERCP and MRCP is 90.6% and the large common bile duct has been mentioned as a factor for MRCP to overlook the bile duct stones.

MRCP has a low diagnostic value compared to EUS in a patient with dilated CBD having small sized stones. Scheiman and his colleagues [29] investigated and compared the cost and clinical efficacy of EUS and MRCP done 24 hours before the ERCP procedure. The authors identified EUS as the best cost-effective modality to prevent unnecessary ERCP. Thus, this will protect patients from potential complications of ERCP. Furthermore, 20% of bile duct stones smaller than 8 mm and detected by MRCP were found to pass spontaneously into the duodenum until the time comes for an ERCP procedure. Thus, EUS will reliably help us to give final decision to do ERCP or not. Another advantage of EUS is its applicability on bed side for patients warded in intensive care units. Additionally, in patients with normal gall bladder evaluation on percutaneous USG, EUS can detect sludge in the gall bladder in the setting of ABP. We can also use a quick EUS examination performed within 72 hours of hospitalization to decide if patients can be discharged early from the hospital. This strategy can decrease the health expanses as well. Thus, it seems very rational to increase cost effectivity of caring for ABP patients by provoking the motivation of ERCP physicians to get learn how to do EUS and vice versa [25–27].

4. First 72 hours treatment steps according to the International Guideliness

Severe cases with ABP should be hospitalized in spesific centers having MRCP, ERCP and preferably EUS facilities under the control of a team of physicians consisted of gastroenterologist, pancreatobiliary surgeon and invasive radiologist [30–35]. First, the severity of AP in accordance with the international scoring models must be determined and the patient's co-morbidities should be recorded. Thereafter, these patients should be vigorously hydrated to prevent the collapse of pancreatic circulation. Indeed, we will especially emphasize aggressive fluid replacement therapy in these patients in the first 3 days of admission with patients with AP. This issue is also very important for the prophylaxis of post-ERCP pancreatitis [36].

A meticiluos fluid replacement within this very 24 hours limits pancreatitis by correcting the hypovolemia and organ hypoperfusion, hinders local and systemic complications of AP by decreasing Systemic Inflammatory Response Syndrome (SIRS) and associated multiorgan failure and lowers inhospital mortality. This helps to improve the general status of the patient and decreases the risks of further invasive procedures like ERCP in these circumstance. During the first 24 hours, iv crystalloid and or colloid solutions can be given [30–35, 37, 38]. Although a retrospective study depicted no difference between ringer lactate (RL) and normal saline (SF) infusion with regard to the severity and complications of pancreatitis [39], there are vast data from the experimental and clinical studies supporting the benefits of RL; such as RL infusion hampers hyperchloremic acidosis and other metabolic complications of AP and by improvinng intraparenchymal pH status, RL infusion inhibits zymogen activation and worsening of AP [40, 41]. For these reasons, RL has been suggested by many international guidelines as first choice to be used as fluid therapy in these patients with AP [30–36]. In the absence of heart and kidney failure, RL infusion at 5–10 ml/kg/hour dose within the first 24 hours is recommended to these patients as targeted fluid therapy. By this way, we aim to get normal hemodynamic parameters, urine output 0.5–1 ml/kg/hour and hematocrit value as between 35–44%. However, we need to be scrupulous to avoid hypervolemia in elderly patients during fluid recesutation. Therefore, it is important to limit the dose to 5 to 10 ml/kg/hour as more than 10 ml/kg/hr. infusion rate has been associated with mehcanical ventilation, abdominal compartment syndorme and increased mortality [42].

5. ERCP when and to whom in ABP?

Before 1978 when Classen [43] first did ERCP and endoscopic sphincterotomy in acute pancreatitis, ERCP was considered as contraindicated in AP. Thereafter, this dogma has changed by Safrany and his collegeus [44] who did ERCP in 15 cases with ABP in 1980. They detected impacted stone at AV in 8 patients and in 7 of them, they showed choledochal stone and removed the stones in all the patients. None of the patients developed any complications and discharged withn a short period after ERCP procedure. After 1980, case series have been reported in this area and first randomized controlled study about this subject was published by Neoptolemos and his collegues in 1986 [3]. In 1993, Fan and et al. [45] published a report in which they investigated the effects of early ERCP on progression of AP. The authors showed that early ERCP was useful only in patients with biliary sepsis compared to conservative group if there is an existing biliary pathology both in mild and severe cases of AP. However, early ERCP did not introduce declined morbidity and mortality when all other etiologies of AP had been included in the study cohort.

Nonetheless, many complications associated with ERCP have been reported in the following years and when and to whom ERCP questions became subject to many researches. ERCP and endoscopic sphinceratomy can make the situation worse in a patient with AP since therapautic ERPC had been reported to have 10% morbidity and 0.1% mortality rates [46, 47]. Additioanlly in patients with AP, there is potential risk of technical failure in ERCP procedure due to edema in the AV and duodenum itself.

For this reason, both the timing of ERCP and detrmining the correct patient who needs this procedure carry the utmost importance. In 2013, International Pancreas Union and American Pancreas Union published together 'the management guideliness of AP' and the suggestions about biliary system problems were written as follows [31]:

1. "ERCP is not indicated in predicted mild biliary pancreatitis without cholangitis. (GRADE 1A, strong agreement). ERCP is probably not indicated in predicted severe biliary pancreatitis without cholangitis (GRADE 1B, strong

agreement). ERCP is probably indicated in biliary pancreatitis with common bile duct obstruction (GRADE 1C,strong agreement) ERCP is indicated in patients with biliary pancreatitis and cholangitis (GRADE 1B, strong agreement)

2. Urgent ERCP (<24 hrs) is required in patients with acute cholangitis. Currently, there is no evidence regarding the optimal timing of ERCP in patients with biliary pancreatitis without cholangitis.(GRADE 2C, strong agreement)

3. MRCP and EUS may prevent a proportion of ERCPs that would otherwise be performed for suspected common bile duct stones in patients with biliary pancreatitis who do not have cholangitis, without influencing the clinical course. EUS is superior to MRCP in excluding the presence of small (<5 mm) gallstones. MRCP is less invasive, less operator-dependent and probably more widely available than EUS. Therefore, in clinical practice there is no clear superiority for either MRCP or EUS.(GRADE 2C, strong agreement)"

Therefore, we will discuss the subject of bliary tree management in patients with AP as subtitiles; 1-Mild pancreatitis in the absence of cholangitis and persistent cholestasis. 2- Severe pancreatitis in the absence of cholangitis and persistent cholestasis 3- Acute pancreatitis together with the presence of cholangitis and persistent cholestasis. We will also discuss; 4- U-ERCP versus E-ERCP and 5-the role of elective ERCP 3 days after patient's admission to prevent recurrence of AP.

5.1 ERCP in patients without cholangitis or persistent cholestasis

The first randomized controlled trial in this field is published by Neoptolemus et al. in 1986 [3]. No relationship was found related to pancreatitis complications and mortality between the conservative treatment group and the ERCP group in mild acute biliary pancreatitis patients in this study and in the meta-analysis which contains 4 randomized controlled studies of Sharma et al. [48]. The patients were stratified by the severity of pancreatitis in the study of Burstow et al. [49] but the patients with or without cholangitis were not analyzed separately and eventually, a strong tendency to decrease pancreatitis complications has been suggested in patients with mild acute biliary pancreatitis, although this is not statistically significant (OR 0.67; 95% CI, 0.43, 1.03; P = 0.06). Another meta-analysis of 5 randomized controlled studies including 702 patients, which compared the conservative treatment and E-ERCP in acute biliary pancreatitis patients by Morietti et al. [50] showed no effect on pancreatitis complications (1.8% (95% CI -5.6% to 9.3%); p = 0.6). Since there is no mortality in patients with mild pancreatitis, a comparison could not be made in this regard. Petrov et al. [51] did not demonstrate any statistically significant difference between the E-ERCP group and the conservative treatment group in terms of reducing complications of pancreatitis in neither mild nor severe acute pancreatitis in their meta-analysis of 5 randomized controlled studies including 717 patients. A systematic review by Geenen et al. that published in Pancreatology in 2013 [52] examined the guidelines and meta-analysis in this field till then, reported that U or E-ERCP±ES had no place in mild acute biliary pancreatitis. As we do in our clinical practice, Elective ERCP (EL-ERCP) might be performed before the cholecystectomy only in case, the stuck stones in AV have escaped back into the choledoc and if this is proved by MRCP or EUS.

As a result, there is consensus that U or E-ERCP±ES is not indicated in mild acute biliary pancreatitis without cholangitis [31, 33–35].

5.2 Emergency ERCP in severe acute biliary patients without cholangitis or persistent cholestasis

ERCP in acute biliary pancreatitis is still a controversial issue, and there no consensus about it. As mentioned before, clinical and animal studies showed that if the biliary obstruction is not terminated within 48 hours, the pathology progresses to necrosis and then organ failure occurs. Therefore, the first studies demonstrated that U or E-ERCP decreased the mortality and morbidity in severe acute pancreatitis patients compared to the control group [53]. In 1997, Fölsch et al. [54] reported that especially deaths due to respiratory failure were more common in the E-ERCP group than the control group in their randomized controlled trial about the role of E-ERCP in acute biliary pancreatitis. The APEC study [4] that includes 232 patients from 26 centers published in July 2020 compared U-ERCP and conservative treatment, and this study changed the paradigm. Besides, acute biliary pancreatitis patients with cholangitis excluded from the APEC study and no significant difference demonstrated between two groups in regard of local or systemic complications of pancreatitis. Whereas, the cholangitis and recurrent attacks of pancreatitis were more common in the U-ERCP group than the conservative treatment group. This is because the criteria for persistent cholestasis or cholangitis were fever, serum bilirubin levels greater than 2.3 mg / dl, commom bile duct width greater than 8 millimeters in patients younger than 75 years and 1 centimeter in patients older than 75 years, and the presence of stones in common bile duct in this study. Another cause of these findings were that it was unclear whether MRCP or EUS, which are the most sensitive methods in detecting stones in choledoc, were performed or not.

Some conflicting results were obtained in the meta-analysis of randomized controlled trials about the role of emergency ERCP in acute biliary pancreatitis, according to the including and excluding criteria of the involved randomized controlled trials and whether subgroup analysis is done or not. Petrov et al. [55] published a meta-analysis in 2008 including 7 randomized controlled trials with 450 patients about the effects of E-ERCP on acute biliary pancreatitis without cholangitis, and they indicated that emergency ERCP has no effect on local complications of pancreatitis in neither mild nor severe pancreatitis. Van Santvoort et al. [56] compared E-ERCP with conservative treatment in patients with and without cholangitis in their randomized controlled trial and demonstrated that in patients without cholestasis, ERCP (29/75 patients: 39%) was not associated with reduced complications (45% vs. 41%, P = 0.814, multivariate adjusted OR: 1.36; 95% CI: 0.49–3.76; P = 0.554) or mortality (14% vs. 17%, P = 0.754, multivariate adjusted OR: 0.78; 95% CI: 0.19–3.12, P = 0.734).

A meta-analysis by Tse et al. [1] which contains 5 randomized controlled studies, indicated that unweighted pooled mortality rates for participants were 9.6% in the early routine ERCP strategy and 4.9% in the early conservative management strategy in patients without cholangitis. Three years after this meta-analysis, Burstow et al. [49] analyzed 11 RCTs consisting of 1314 patients (conservative management = 662, ERCP = 652). There was a near significant decrease in mortality for the ERCP group compared with conservatively managed patients with severe pancreatitis [odds ratio (OR) 0.45; 95% confidence interval (CI), 0.19, 1.09; P = 0.08]. In patients with mild pancreatitis, mortality results were comparable for both groups (OR 0.66; 95% CI, 0.02, 28.75; P = 0.83). Overall complications were significantly reduced in the ERCP group in severe pancreatitis patients (OR 0.32; 95% CI, 0.17,0.61; P = 0.00). The authors' comments about this meta-analysis are as follows: this meta-analysis demonstrates a significant decrease in complications in patients with severe ABP managed with early ERCP/ES compared with conservative management. As far as the mortality is concerned, no significant decrease was observed in mortality even in severe ABP patients treated with early ERCP/ES.

The meta-analysis and systematic review about the comparison of E-ERCP and conservative treatment in acute biliary pancreatitis by Coutinho et al. [57] reported that; the pain and fever resolved in a shorter time, the hospitalization time was shorter with reduced complications and hospital costs were lower in the E-ERCP group than the conservative treatment group. Uy et al. [58] performed a meta-analysis including 2 randomized controlled trials that compares the E-ERCP (n = 177) and the conservative treatment (n = 163) in acute biliary pancreatitis. This meta-analysis revealed low mortality rates for both mild and severe pancreatitis in the ERCP group (RR = 1.92, 95% CI: 0.86–4.32) whereas the morbidity rates were similar in both groups (RR = 0.95, 95% CI: 0.74–1.22). Moretti et al. [50] demonstrated that ERCP had no effect on complications in mild pancreatitis however, ERCP reduced the complications in severe pancreatitis but it did not have any effect on mortality rates in their meta-analysis including 5 prospective randomized trials with 702 patients. Geenen et al. [52] preformed a review including 12 international guidelines and 8 meta-analysis. Although 3 meta-analysis and 1 guideline recommended against ERCP in acute biliary pancreatitis, 7 out of 11 guidelines recommended routine E-ERCP in severe acute biliary pancreatitis regardless of the presence of cholangitis, and they agreed on the lack of consensus about routine E-ERCP in severe acute biliary pancreatitis. However, the 4 main international guidelines that we evaluated (2 out of them belonged the same group but published at different times) recommended against the emergency ERCP in acute biliary pancreatitis without cholangitis because it did not significantly reduce mortality and morbidity compared to the conservative treatment group [31, 33–35]. Contrary to these guidelines, another guideline of the United Kingdom publishe in 2005 [32] has controversial suggestions about E-ERCP in severe acute biliary pancreatitis without cholangitis as; "*Urgent therapeutic endoscopic retrograde cholangiopancreatography (ERCP) should be performed in patients with acute pancreatitis of suspected or proven gall stone etiology who satisfy the criteria for predicted or actual severe pancreatitis, or when there is cholangitis, jaundice, or a dilated common bile duct.* ".

Because of the lack of statically significant data about the reduction in local and systemic complications or mortality rates of pancreatitis by emergency ERCP in severe acute biliary pancreatitis from many RCTs and meta-analyzes until to date, international guidelines referring to these results indicated that U- or E-ERCP have no benefit in every patient with severe acute biliary pancreatitis unless cholangitis is present. The ESGE guideline published in 2018 [33] explains why ERCP should not be performed in a patient with severe pancreatitis without cholangitis: "*A possible explanation why urgent ERCP with sphincterotomy within 24 h did not show an advantage over conservative treatment could be that the opportunity to positively influence the disease course had already passed at the time of the ERCP despite the fact that it was performed early. Animal models have shown that trypsinogen activation within the pancreas occurs within10 min after chemically inducing pancreatitis. It is well known that most bile duct stones in patients with gallstone pancreatitis cause only temporary obstruction and pass spontaneously into the duodenum. This temporary obstruction already initiates pancreatitis and data from animal models show that this includes intrapancreatic trypsin activation, rupturing of vacuoles releasing active trypsin, and pancreatic autodigestion. In the current trial, urgent ERCP was done after a median*

29 h after onset of symptoms and common bile duct stones were found in 43% of patients. Even this narrow time window might already be too long to prevent pancreatitis from deteriorating by performing an urgent ERCP with sphincterotomy".

5.3 Emergency ERCP in acute biliary patients with cholangitis or persistent cholestasis

Certainly, biliopancreatic obstruction should be resolved immediately in patients with cholangitis or persistent cholestasis. The most effective method of this is undoubtedly the removal of stone or sludge that caused the obstruction by performing ERCP and ES [59]. The first study in this area was performed by Neoptolemos et al. and it demonstrated that E-ERCP and ES was the most useful method in acute biliary pancreatitis with cholangitis and cholangitis without pancreatitis [60]. Van Santvoort et al. [56] performed a study about the efficiency of ERCP in acute pancreatitis patient with or without cholestasis and findings as follows: In patients with cholestasis, ERCP (52/78 patients: 67%), as compared with conservative treatment, was associated with fewer complications (25% vs. 54%, P = 0.020, multivariate adjusted odds ratio [OR]: 0.35, 95% confidence interval [CI]: 0.13–0.99, P = 0.049). This included fewer patients with >30% pancreatic necrosis (8% vs. 31%, P = 0.010). Mortality was nonsignificantly lower after ERCP (6% vs. 15%, P = 0.213, multivariate adjusted OR: 0.44, 95% CI: 0.08–2.28, P = 0.330).

Tse et al. [1] performed a meta-analysis which included 5 randomized controlled trials with 644 participants with cholangitis and reported mortality rates, comprising a total of 200 participants in the early routine ERCP strategy and 215 in the early conservative management strategy. Unweighted pooled mortality rates for participants were 1.0% for the early routine ERCP strategy and 6.9% in the early conservative management strategy. In the trials that included participants with cholangitis, the early routine ERCP strategy significantly reduced mortality compared to the early conservative management strategy (RR 0.20, 95% CI 0.06 to 0.68; P = 0.010).

5.4 U-ERCP or E-ERCP in acute biliary pancreatitis with cholangitis or persistent cholestasis?

There is no consensus on timing of ERCP in the literature. In most publications, the ERCP preformed within 72 hours after the symptom onset is called emergency ERCP, but the emergency ERCP timing could be defined as within 48 hours in some other publications. Additionally, the ERCP which is performed within 72 hours named as U-ERCP in some publications. The only trial that compares the timing of ERCP (within 24 hours versus within 24–72 hours) in acute biliary pancreatitis is performed by Lee et al. [2]. Patients with acute biliary pancreatitis but without cholangitis was excluded retrospectively in this study, and they compared U-ERCP and E-ERCP in acute biliary pancreatitis. No significant difference was found in the total length of hospitalization or procedural-related complications, in patients with biliary pancreatitis and a bile duct obstruction without cholangitis, according to the timing of ERCP (< 24 h vs. 24–72 h). Although the definition is not U-ERCP, in one of Fan et al.'s studies [45] the ERCP which is performed within 24 hours is defined as E-ERCP and there was no significant difference between the ERCP group and the conservative treatment group in terms of local and systemic complications of pancreatitis whereas hospitalization time was a little shorter in the E-ERCP group. With these results, it was demonstrated that performing U-ERCP within 24 hours did not change the pancreatitis course, supporting the study of Lee et al. [2]. When considering the course of acute biliary pancreatitis, naming the ERCP performed within 24 hours as "URGENT" and the ERCP within 24–72 hours as "EARLY" by

Lee et al. is the most appropriate definition [2]. When the literature and international guidelines are reviewed, ERCP is recommended to the acute biliary pancreatitis within 24 hours if the cholangitis is present and within 72 hours if the biliary obstruction is present, instead of this definition.

Although the naming does not resemble, recommendation of ESGE in this respect is as follows: "*ESGE recommends urgent (≤ 24 hours) ERCP and biliary drainage in patients with acute biliary pancreatitis combined with cholangitis. Strong recommendation, high quality of evidence. ERCP should be performed within 72 hours in patients with ongoing biliary obstruction. Weak recommendation, moderate quality evidence. It should not be performed in patients with acute biliary pancreatitis and neither cholangitis or ongoing bile duct obstruction. Weak recommendation, moderate quality evidence*" [33]. According to our clinical experience; although there is a need for randomized prospective trials on this subject, the absence of difference between performing the ERCP within 24 hours or within 24–72 hours leads to escape gastroenterologist or endoscopists from the regression of performing ERCP within 24 hours in a rush and off-duty, which is believed to be the reason of high rates of complications such as aggrevation of pancreatitis, possible bilioportal reflux in patients with cholangitis during ERCP, bacteriemia or systemic complications (i.e., organ failure) by depriving the patient's opportunity to receive extensive fluid therapy and broad-spectrum antibiotics within the most important 24 hours for the complications.

5.5 Elective ERCP to prevent pancreatitis recurrence

Early laparoscopic or open cholecystectomy as soon as AP recovers completely is the only proven treatment modality to prevent recurrence of ABP. Index cholecystectomy is defined as cholecystectomy applied during the same hospitalization period of ABP and interval cholcystectonmy is cholecystectomy performed 6 weeks after patient's recovery from AP [61].

Sinha and colleagues [61] reported that index cholecystectomy in a case suitable for surgery has similar results with elective cholecystectomy in a patient without AP and they also reported significant difficulty to do dissection during interval cholecystectomy. In 2019, Fu-ping Zhung and colleagues [62] published a meta-analysis of 19 studies enrolling 2639 who underwent index or interval cholecystectomy. They noted that there was no differences with ragard to intraoperative and postoperative complications, duration of operation and the rates of open cholecystectomy. However, index cholecystectomy cases had lesser hospitalization period, lower biliary complications due to surgery and lesser rates of ERCP.

In cases with severe pancreatitis, most of the time it is impracticable to perform index cholcystectomy. Therefore, interval cholcystectomy is obligatory in these cases. Infortunately, these patients reamit with AP attacks and ot biliary complications during this 6 weeks period. Thus some authors offer ERCP and endoscopic sphincteratomy to prevent AP recurrences and or biliary complications to ocur during this time period [63, 64].

In a retrospective study comparing index cholecystectomy and post ERCP/ES plus interval cholecystectomy, both group of patients did not reveal mortality. Only 2 patients (%5) developed AP recurrences and acute cholecystitis and hospitalized. The authors suggested that ERCP/ES is highly successful to prevent recurrences in patients with severe ABP who can not undergo index cholecystectomy. ES and interval cholecystectomy in severe ABP is considered a reasonable alternative to an index cholecystectomy in patients with severe ABP [64].

Another report by Dedemadi and his colleagues [65] published in 2016 noted that ERCP and ES in cases with AP who can not undergo cholecystectomy developed biliary events 0%–28.6%, recurrent pancreatitis 0%–8.2%, mortality 3%–4.7%. Other cases under conservative treatment had biliary events 9.4%–14.3%, recurrent pancreatitis 12%–23%, mortality 3.9%. Statistical evaluation showed that ERCP and ES group had significanly less biliary complications and less recurrent pancreatitis with no difference in mortality compared to conservative treatment group. The conservative group consisted of patients who were elderly persons with multiple comorbidites and complications of AP. These conditions may be responsible for similar mortality rates in both groups. Nevertheless, because of high rates of biliary events and pancreatitis in the ERPC/ES group, this approach should be reserved only for patients not suitaable for cholecystectomy.

The advice of IAP/APA about timing od cholecystectomy in a case with ABP is as follows [31]:

5.5.1 "Timing of cholecystectomy (or endoscopic sphincterotomy)

1. *Cholecystectomy during index admission for mild biliary pancreatitis appears safe and is recommended. Interval cholecystectomy after mild biliary pancreatitis isassociated with a substantial risk of readmission for recurrent biliary events, especially recurrent biliary pancreatitis. (GRADE 1C, strong agreement).*

2. *Cholecystectomy should be delayed in patients with peripancreatic collections until the collections either resolve or if they persist beyond 6 weeks, at which time cholecystectomy can be performed safely. (GRADE 2C, strong agreement).*

3. *In patients with biliary pancreatitis who have undergone sphincterotomy and are fit for surgery, cholecystectomy is advised, because ERCP and sphincterotomy prevent recurrence of biliary pancreatitis but not gallstone related gallbladder disease, i.e. biliary colic and cholecystitis. (GRADE 2B, strong agreement)".*

Moreover, If we consider surgery for pancreatic cystic collections, pseudocysyt and or walled off necrosis, it should be performed at the same time with cholecystectomy [65].

6. Conclusion

We want to finish with the conclsuive statement made by ESGE [35]; *"In conclusion, urgent ERCP with sphincterotomy did not reduce the composite endpoint of major complications or mortality in patients with predicted severe gallstone pancreatitis, compared with conservative treatment. These findings support a conservative strategy with an ERCP indicated only in patients with cholangitis or persistent cholestasis. With this conservative strategy, about two-thirds of patients did not need to undergo ERCP".* In the presence of cholangitis, ERCP as E-ERCP should be done only after hemodynamic stabilisation and relieved organ hipoperfusion with aggressive fluid replacement and antibiotic treatment within the first 24 hours, Elective ERCP to prevent ABP attacks is suggested only for patients unsuitable for an choecystectomy procedure.

Author details

Ülkü Saritaş[1]* and Yücel Üstündağ[2]

1 Emeritus Professor, Suleyman Demirel University, Turkey

2 Bülent Ecevit University, Zonguldak, Turkey

*Address all correspondence to: saritasulku@yahoo.com

References

[1] Tse F,Yuan Y.Early routine endoscopic retrograde cholangio pancreatographystrategy versus early conservative management strategy in acute gallstone pancreatitis. Cochrane Database Syst Rev 2012 May 16;(5):CD009779.doi: 10.1002/14651858. CD009779.pub

[2] Lee HS, Chung MJ, Park YJ, Bang S, Park SW, Song SY, Jae Bock Chun BJ. Urgent endoscopic retrograde cholangiopancreatography is not superior to early ERCP in acute biliary pancreatitis with biliary obstruction without cholangitis PLoS One. 2018;13(2):e0190835.Published online 2018 Feb 5.doi:10.1371/journal. pone.0190835

[3] Neoptolemos JP, London N, Slater ND, Carr-Locke DL, Fossard DP, Moosa AR A prospective study of in the diagnosis and treatment of gallstone acute pancreatitis A rational and safe approach to management Arch Surg. 1986 Jun;121(6):697-702

[4] Schepers NJ, Hallensleben NDL et all. Urgent endoscopic retrograde cholangiopancreatography with sphincterotomy versus conservative treatment in severe acute gallstone pancreatitis (APEC):A multicentre randomised controlled trial. Lancet 2020, 396 (10245);167-176

[5] Santos JS, Kemp R, Ardengh JC, Jr JE. Conservative management of cholestasis with and without fever in acute biliary pancreatitis. World J Gastrointest Surg. 2012;4:55-61.

[6] Baillie J. Should urgent ERCP be performed in patients with acute biliary pancreatitis without acute cholangitis?Nat Clin Pract Gastroenterol Hepatol. 2008 Sep;5(9):484-5

[7] Hirano T, Manabe T. A possible mechanism for gallstone pancreatitis: repeated short- term pancreaticobiliary duct obstruction with exocrine stimulation in rats. Proc Soc Exp Biol Med. 1993;202:246-252.

[8] Runzi M, Saluja A, Lerch MM, Dawra R, Nishino H, Steer ML. Early ductal decompression prevents the progression of biliary pancreatitis: an experimental study in the opossum. Gastroenterology. 1993;105:157-164

[9] Senninger N, Moody FG, Coelho JC, Van Buren DH. The role of biliary obstruction in the pathogenesis of acute pancreatitis in the opossum. Surgery. 1986;99:688-693

[10] Frossard JL, Hadengue A, Amouyal G, Choury A, Marty O, Giostra E, Sivignon F, Sosa L, Amouyal P. Choledocholithiasis: a prospective study of spontaneous common bile duct stone migration. Gastrointest Endosc. 2000;51:175-179

[11] Acosta JM, Rubio Galli OM, Rossi R, Chinellato AV, Pellegrini CA. Effect of duration of ampullary gallstone obstruction on severity of lesions of acute pancreatitis. J Am Coll Surg. 1997;184: 499-50

[12] Acosta JM, Katkhouda N, Debian KA, Groshen SG, Tsao-Wei DD, Berne TV. Early ductal decompression versus conservative management for gallstone pancreatitis with ampullary obstruction: a prospective randomized clinical trial. Ann Surg. 2006 Jan;243(1):33-40

[13] Cavdar F, Yildar M, Tellioglu G, Kara M, Tilki M, Titiz MI. Controversial issues in biliary pancreatitis: when should we perform MRCP and ERCP? Pancreatology. 2014;14: 411-414

[14] Acosta JM, Ronzano GD, Pellegrini CA. Ampullary obstruction monitoring in acute gallstone

pancreatitis: a safe, accurate, and reliable method to detect pancreatic ductal obstruction. Am J Gastroenterol. 2000 Jan;95(1):122-127

[15] Paloyan D, Simonowitz D, Skinner DB. The timing of biliary tract operations in patients with pancreatitis associated with gallstones. Surg Gynecol Obstet. 1975;141:737-739

[16] Frei GJ, Frei VT, Thirlby RC, McClelland RN. Biliary pancreatitis: clinical presentation and surgical management. Am J Surg. 1986;151:170-175.

[17] Chang L, Lo SK, Stabile BE, Lewis RJ, de Virgilio C. Gallstone pancreatitis: a prospective study on the incidence of cholangitis and clinical predictors of retained common bile duct stones. Am J Gastroenterol. 1998;93:527-531.

[18] Cohen ME, Slezak L, Wells CK, Andersen DK, Topazian M. Prediction of bile duct stones and complications in gallstone pancreatitis using early laboratory trends. Am J Gastroenterol. 2001;96:3305-3311.

[19] Cetta F Gallstone pancreatitis, associated cholangitis, clinical predictors of persistent common duct stones, and ERCP or endoscopic sphincterotomy. Am J Gastroenterol. 1998; 93:493-6

[20] Anderloni A, Ballarè M, Pagliarulo M, Conte D, Galeazzi M, Orsello M, Andorno S Del Piano M. Prospective evaluation of early endoscopic ultrasonography for triage in suspected choledocholithiasis: results from a large single centre series. Dig Liver Dis. 2014;46:335-339. 3 1;154(4):1096-101.

[21] Ainsworth AP, Rafaelsen SR, Wamberg PA, Durup J, Pless TK, Mortensen MB. Is there a difference in diagnostic accuracy and clinical impact between endoscopic ultrasonography and magnetic resonance cholangiopancreatography? Endoscopy. 2003;35:1029-1032.

[22] Romagnuolo J, Bardou M, Rahme E, Joseph L, Reinhold C, Barkun AN. Magnetic resonance cholangiopancreatography: a meta-analysis of test performance in suspected biliary disease. Ann Intern Med. 2003;139:547-557.

[23] Anderloni A, Repici A. Role and timing of endoscopy in acute biliary pancreatitis World J Gastroenterol. 2015; 21: 11205-11208.

[24] De Lisi S, Leandro G, Buscarini E. Endoscopic ultrasonography versus endoscopic retrograde cholangiopancreatography in acute biliary pancreatitis: a systematic review. Eur J Gastroenterol Hepatol. 2011;23:367-374.

[25] Tse F, Liu L, Barkun AN, Armstrong D, Moayyedi P. EUS: a meta-analysis of test performance in suspected choledocholithiasis. Gastrointest Endosc. 2008;67:235-244

[26] Benjaminov F, Stein A, Lichtman G, Pomeranz I, Konikoff FM. Consecutive versus separate sessions of endoscopic ultrasound (EUS) and endoscopic retrograde cholangiopancreatography (ERCP) for symptomatic choledocholithiasis. Surg Endosc. 2013;27:2117-2121.

[27] Savides TJ. EUS-guided ERCP for patients with intermediate probability for choledocholithiasis: is it time for all of us to start doing this? Gastrointest Endosc. 2008;67:669-672.

[28] Moon JH, Cho YD, Cha SW, Cheon YK, Ahn HC, Kim YS, Kim YS, Lee JS, Lee MS, Lee HK, et al. The detection of bile duct stones in suspected biliary pancreatitis: comparison of MRCP, ERCP, and

intraductal US. Am J Gastroenterol. 2005;100:1051-1057

[29] Scheiman JM, Carlos RC, Barnett JL, Elta GH, Nostrant TT, Chey WD, Francis IR, Nandi PS. Can endoscopic ultrasound or magnetic resonance cholangiopancreatography replace ERCP in patients with suspected biliary disease? A prospective trial and cost analysis. Am J Gastroenterol. 2001;96:2900-2904.

[30] James TW, Crockett SD Management of Acute Pancreatitis in the First 72 hours Curr Opin Gastroenterol. 2018; 34(5): 330-335.

[31] Besselink M, van Santvoort H, Freeman M, et al. Working Group IAP/APA evidence-based guidelines for the management of acute pancreatitis. Pancreatology. 2013;13(4 Suppl 2):e1-15.

[32] UK guidelines for the management of acute pancreatitis Working Party of the British Society of Gastroenterology; Association of Surgeons of Great Britain and Ireland; Pancreatic Society of Great Britain and Ireland; Association of Upper GI Surgeons of Great Britain and Ireland Gut 2005 May;54 Suppl 3(Suppl 3):iii1-9. doi: 10.1136/gut.2004.057026.

[33] Arvanitakis M, Dumonceau JM, Albert J, et al. Endoscopic management of acute necrotizing pancreatitis: European Society of Gastrointestinal Endoscopy (ESGE) evidence-based multidisciplinary guidelines. Endoscopy 2018; 50: 524-46.

[34] Tenner S, Baille J, DeWitt J, Vege SS, American College of G. American College of Gastroenterology guideline: management of acute pancreatitis. Am J Gastroenterol. 2013;108: 1400-1415

[35] Crockett SD, Wani S, Gardner TB, et al. American Gastroenterological Association Institute Guideline on Initial Management of Acute Pancreatitis. Gastroenterology. 2018

[36] Senol A, Saritas U, Demirkan H. Efficacy of intramuscular diclofenac and fluid replacement in prevention of post ERCP pancreatitis. World J Gastroenterol 2009; 15: 3999-4004

[37] Mao EQ, Tang YQ, Fei J, Qin S, Wu J, Li L, et al. Fluid therapy for severe acute pancreatitis in acute response stage. Chin Med J (Engl) 2009;122:169e73.

[38] Mole DJ, Hall A, McKeown D, Garden OJ, Parks RW. Detailed fluid resuscitation profiles in patients with severe acute pancreatitis. HPB (Oxford) 2011;13:51-58.

[39] Lipinski M, Rydzewska-Rosolowska A, Rydzewski A, Rydzewska G. . Fluid resuscitation in acute pancreatitis: Normal saline or lactated Ringer's solution?World J Gastroenterol. 2015 21;21(31):9367-72. doi: 10.3748/wjg.v21.i31.9367

[40] Wu BU, Hwang JQ, Gardner TH, Repas K, Delee R, Yu S, et al. Lactated Ringer's solution reduces systemic inflammation compared with saline in patients with acute pancreatitis. Clin Gastroenterol Hepatol 2011;9:710-717.

[41] Perner A, Haase N, Guttormsen AB, Tenhunen J, Klemenzson G, Aneman A,et al. Hydroxyethyl starch 130/0.42 versus Ringer's acetate in severe sepsis.N Engl J Med 2012;367:124-134

[42] Mao EQ, Fei J, Peng YB, Huang J, Tang YQ, Zhang SD. Rapid hemodilution isassociated with increased sepsis and mortality among patients with severe acute pancreatitis. Chin Med J (Engl) 2010;123:1639e44.

[43] Classen M., Ossenberg, F. W., Wurbs, D., et al.: Pancreatitis-an indication for endoscopic papillotomy? Endoscopy, 10:223, 1978.

[44] Safrany, L, Neuhaus, B., Krause, S., et al.: Endoskopische Papillotomie bei

akuter bilier Pankreatitis. Dtsch. Med. Wschr., 105:115, 1980

[45] Fan ST, Lai EC, Mok FP, Lo CM, Zheng SS, Wong J. Early treatment of acute biliary pancreatitis by endoscopic papillotomy. N Engl J Med. 1993;328: 228-232.

[46] Loperfido S, Angelini G, Benedetti G, Chilovi F, Costan F, De Berardinis F, De Bernardin M, Ederle A, Fina P, Fratton *A. major* early complications from diagnostic and therapeutic ERCP: a prospective multicenter study. Gastrointest Endosc. 1998;48:1-10.

[47] Cotton PB, Lehman G, Vennes J, Geenen JE, Russell RC, Meyers WC, Liguory C, Nickl N. Endoscopic sphincterotomy complications and their management: an attempt at consensus. Gastrointest Endosc. 1991;37:383-393

[48] Sharma VK, Howden CW. Metaanalysis of randomized controlled trials of endoscopic retrograde cholangiography and endoscopicsphincterotomy for the treatment of acute biliary pancreatitis. Am J Gastroenterol. 1999;94:3211-3214.

[49] Burstow MJ, Rossita M. Yunus RM, Hossain B, Khan S ET ALL Meta-Analysis of Early Endoscopic Retrograde Cholangiopancreatography (ERCP) ± Endoscopic Sphincterotomy (ES) Versus Conservative Management for Gallstone Pancreatitis (GSP) Surg Laparosc Endosc Percutan Tech 2015;25:185-203)

[50] Moretti A, Papi C, Aratari A, et al. Is early endoscopic retrograde cholangiopancreatography useful in the management of acute biliary pancreatitis? A meta-analysis of randomized controlled trials. Dig Liver Dis. 2008;40:379-385

[51] Petrov MS, Uchugina AF, Kukosh MV. Does endoscopic retrograde cholangiopancreatography reduce the risk of local pancreatic complications in acute pancreatitis? A systematic review and metaanalysis. Surg Endosc. 2008;22:2338-2343

[52] van Geenen EJ, van Santvoort HC, Besselink MG, van der Peet DL, van Erpecum KJ, Fockens P, Mulder CJ, Bruno MJ Lack of consensus on the role of endoscopic retrograde cholangiography in acute biliary pancreatitis in published meta-analyses and guidelines: a systematic review Pancreas 2013 Jul;42(5):774-80

[53] Neoptolemos JP, Carr-Locke DL, London NJ, Bailey IA, James D, Fossard DP. Controlled trial of urgent endoscopic retrograde cholangiopancreatography and endoscopic sphincterotomy versus conservative treatment for acute pancreatitis due to gallstones. Lancet 1988; 2: 979-983

[54] Folsch UR, Nitsche R, Ludtke R, Hilgers RA, Creutzfeldt W. Early ERCP and papillotomy compared with conservative treatment for acute biliary pancreatitis. The German Study Group on Acute Biliary Pancreatitis. N Engl J Med. 1997;336: 237-24

[55] Petrov MS, van Santvoort HC, Besselink MG, et al. Early endoscopic retrograde cholangiopancreatography versus conservative management in acute biliary pancreatitis without cholangitis: a meta-analysis of randomized trials. Ann Surg. 2008;247:250-257.

[56] van Santvoort HC, Besselink MG, de Vries AC, Boermeester MA, Fischer K, Bollen TL, et al. Early endoscopic retrograde cholangiopancreatography in predicted severe acute biliary pancreatitis: a prospective multicenter study. Ann Surg. 2009;250: 68-75Roesch W, Ludwig Demling L. Endoscopic Management of Pancreatitis Surgical Clinics of North America-Yo!. 62, No.5, October 1982

[57] Coutinho, Lara M. de A.; Bernardo, Wanderley M.; Rocha, Rodrigo S.; More Early Endoscopic Retrograde Cholangiopancreatography Versus Conservative Treatment in Patients With Acute Biliary Pancreatitis: Systematic Review and Meta-analysis of Randomized Controlled Trials Pancreas 2018, 47(4):444-453

[58] Uy MC, Daez ML, Sy PP, et al. Early ERCP in acute gallstone pancreatitis without cholangitis: a meta-analysis. JOP.2009;10:299-305

[59] Kapetanos DJ. ERCP in acute biliary pancreatitis. World J Gastrointest Endosc. 2010;2: 25-28R

[60] Neoptolemos JP, Carr-Locke DL, Leese T, James D. Acute cholangitis in association with acute pancreatitis: incidence,clinical features and outcome in relation to ERCP and endoscopic sphincterotomy. Br J Surg 1987; 74: 1103-1106

[61] Sinha R Early laparoscopic cholecystectomy in acute biliary pancreatitis: the optimal choice? HPB (Oxford). 2008 Oct 1; 10(5): 332-335. doi: 10.1080/13651820802247078

[62] Fu-ping Zhong, Kai Wang, Xue-qin Tan, Jian Nie, Wen-feng Huang, Xiao-fang Wang The optimal timing of laparoscopic cholecystectomy in patients with mild gallstone pancreatitis: A meta-analysis Medicine (Baltimore) 2019 Oct; 98(40): e17429. Published online 2019 Oct 4.

[63] Sanjay P, Yeeting S, Whigham C, Judson H, Polignano FM, Tait SI. Endoscopic sphincterotomy and interval cholecystectomy are reasonable alternatives to index cholecystectomy in severe acute gallstone pancreatitis (GSP) Surg Endosc 2008 Aug;22(8):1832-7. doi: 10.1007/s00464-007-9710-1. Epub 2007 Dec 11

[64] Emad Q, Rushikesh S; Haddad YK. Endoscopic Retrograde Cholangiopancreatography Decreases All-Cause and Pancreatitis Readmissions in Patients With Acute Gallstone Pancreatitis Who Do Not Undergo Cholecystectomy A Nationwide 5-Year Analysis Pancreas 2018, 47: 425-435

[65] Dedemadi G, Nikolopoulos M, Kalaitzopoulos I, Sgourakis G Management of patients after recovering from acute severe biliary pancreatitisWorld J Gastroenterol. 2016 Sep 14; 22(34): 7708-7717. Published online 2016 Sep 14. doi: 10.3748/wjg.v22.i34.770

Chapter 5

Surgical Management of Necrotizing Pancreatitis

Dane Thompson, Siavash Bolourani and Matthew Giangola

Abstract

Pancreatic necrosis is a highly morbid condition. It is most commonly associated with severe, acute pancreatitis, but can also be caused by trauma or chronic pancreatitis. Once diagnosed, management of pancreatic necrosis begins with supportive care, with an emphasis on early, and preferably, enteral nutrition. Intervention for necrosis, sterile or infected, is dictated by patient symptoms and response to conservative management. When possible, intervention should be delayed to allow the necrotic collection to form a capsule. First-line treatment for necrosis is with percutaneous drainage or endoscopic, transmural drainage. These strategies can be effective as monotherapy, but the need for repeated interventions, or for progression to more invasive interventions, is not uncommon. Necrosectomy may be performed using a previously established drainage tract, as in percutaneous endoscopic necrosectomy (PEN), video-assisted retroperitoneal debridement (VARD), and direct endoscopic necrosectomy (DEN). Although outcomes for these minimally-invasive techniques are better than for traditional necrosectomy, both laparoscopic and open techniques remain important for patients with extensive disease that cannot otherwise be adequately treated. This is especially true when pancreatic necrosis is complicated by disconnected pancreatic duct syndrome (DPDS), where necrosectomy remains standard of care.

Keywords: necrotizing pancreatitis, pancreatic necrosis, percutaneous, endoscopic, pancreatectomy, necrosectomy

1. Introduction

Pancreatic necrosis is the presence of nonviable pancreatic parenchyma or peripancreatic fat which may be localized or diffuse. It is classified radiologically according to the Atlanta Criteria as an acute necrotic collection (ANC), which is defined as a non-encapsulated area of necrosis, or as walled-off necrosis (WON), which is encapsulated [1]. Although pancreatic necrosis may result from trauma, malignancy, or chronic pancreatitis, the most common cause is acute pancreatitis; 20% of patients with acute pancreatitis develop necrosis. For patients who develop necrosis, the mortality rate is 15–30% [2]. Surgery has historically been the primary treatment for pancreatic necrosis. However, the superior outcomes associated with new, less invasive techniques have narrowed the scope for surgical intervention. Despite these shifts in practice, surgical care remains an important tool for the treatment of pancreatic necrosis.

2. Diagnosis and conservative management

Although the diagnosis of pancreatitis is generally clinical, the primary diagnostic tool for pancreatic necrosis is the computed tomography (CT) scan. With this modality, normal pancreatic parenchyma is low attenuation, 40–50 Hounsfield units (HU), but increases with contrast to 100–150 HU. In comparison, areas of necrosis remain hypoattenuating, <30 HU [3]. MRI and endoscopic ultrasound are also used, but CT scan is considered to be the gold standard for diagnosis and characterization [4].

Regardless of the presence of necrosis, fluid resuscitation, and early nutritional support are paramount to the treatment of patients with acute pancreatitis. For patients who are able to tolerate enteral nutrition, there is a significant reduction in the rates of infected pancreatic necrosis, multiorgan failure, surgical intervention, and mortality when compared to patients who are given total parenteral nutrition (TPN) [5, 6]. Thus, prior to initiation of TPN, patients should be evaluated for tolerance of oral, nasogastric, and nasojejunal feeding. Route notwithstanding, nutrition should be addressed in the first 24–48 hours of admission for acute pancreatitis [7].

Sterile pancreatic necrosis does not have a specific clinical presentation, but is more common in patients with symptoms lasting more than 48 hours and with concomitant organ failure [8]. The morbidity and mortality associated with pancreatic necrosis is exacerbated by development of infection, which may result of seeding associated with bacteremia, colonic bacterial translocation, or direct contamination from a procedure (e.g. endoscopic retrograde cholangiopancreatography (ERCP) or surgery) [9]. The risk of infection correlates with the degree of necrosis. If more than 30% of the pancreatic parenchyma is necrotic, there is a 22% risk of infection. If 30–50% is necrotic, the risk of infection is 37%. If necrosis exceeds 50%, the risk of infection is 46% [10]. The signs and symptoms of infected pancreatic necrosis are similar to those of other types of infection, including: fever, leukocytosis, and worsening condition with optimal supportive care. Once the necrosis becomes infected, the incidence of organ failure increases, along with the risk of mortality [11].

Differentiating sterile from infected necrosis based on clinical presentation can be difficult. Patients with sterile necrosis can proceed to organ failure in similar fashion to patients with infected necrosis. Infection can be detected non-invasively on CT scan by looking for the presence of gas locules within the area of necrosis, suggesting microbial gas production. However, these findings are not always seen on CT, and fine-needle aspiration (FNA) may be necessary for definitive diagnosis. Multiple FNA aspirates may be required due to the 10% false negative rate of this test [12].

However, proof of infection on radiology or by tissue culture is not necessary to initiate treatment. If infection is strongly suspected due to clinical course, antibiotics are indicated regardless of radiologic or tissue diagnosis. If no antibiotic sensitivities are available from culture results, broad-spectrum antibiotics should be started. Due to the ability to penetrate the necrotic tissue, carbapenems are considered first-line treatment [13]. Prophylactic use of antibiotics has not been shown to impact the rate of developing infected necrosis, systemic complications, mortality, or need for surgical intervention and is not recommended [14–16].

Prior to any invasive management, a patient should be treated with optimal supportive care. This includes fluid resuscitation, nutritional support, and antibiotics, if infection is suspected. The need for invasive management of sterile pancreatic necrosis is rare, especially in acute phase. However intervention may be necessary during the late phase for protracted abdominal pain, obstruction, or, less often, for failure of clinical improvement. Infected necrosis requires invasive intervention more often, both in order to gain source control and in order to resolve other non-infectious symptoms [17].

3. Percutaneous and endoscopic interventions

Although percutaneous and endoscopic interventions have historically been considered temporizing measures, not definitive management, many patients with pancreatic necrosis are successfully treated with these techniques, without need for more invasive therapy. Percutaneous drainage can successfully treat acute necrotizing pancreatitis in more than 50% of patients without need for surgical necrosectomy. The success rate with endoscopic therapy can reach 80% when used in conjunction with DEN [18, 19]. Thus, development of less invasive methods for addressing pancreatic necrosis led to a decrease in the indications for surgical intervention. The choice of intervention, percutaneous or endoscopic, is dependent on the situation, timing, and accessibility of the area of necrosis (**Figure 1**).

Endoscopic management of pancreatic necrosis is performed transmurally, either across the duodenum, for pancreatic head necrosis, or the stomach, for neck or body necrosis. Although technically feasible earlier in the clinical course, endoscopic intervention should be delayed to 4 weeks after onset of symptoms in order for an appropriate capsule to form around the necrotic tissue [20]. In cases where intervention can be delayed until WON form, and the WON is accessible transmurally, this is considered first-line intervention [18].

With or without the aid of endoscopic ultrasound (EUS), a plastic or self-expanding metal stent (SEMS) is placed from the lumen of the duodenum or stomach into the area of WON. In addition to allowing the WON to drain into the

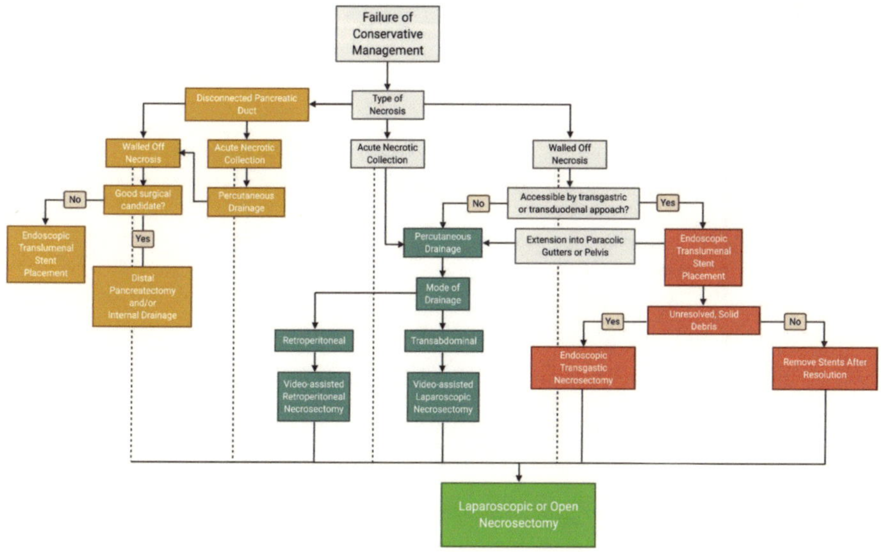

Figure 1.
Flowchart for Management of Pancreatic Necrosis after Failure of conservative management. After failure of conservative management – Supportive care, antibiotics, and nutrition – The appropriate intervention depends on the nature of the necrosis. If it is associated with a disconnected duct, a separate pathway, which ends with distal pancreatectomy, internal drainage, or endoscopic translumenal stent placement, is indicated. If there is no disconnected duct, the correct pathway is dictated by the stage of necrosis, as a nonencapsulated acute necrotic collection or as walled off necrosis. Endoscopic and percutaneous strategies are preferred in each situation, and traditional, laparoscopic or open necrosectomy serves as the final option for patients that fail other management, or in hospitals without resources or staff to perform other procedures.

lumen, these stents also allow access to the area for debridement, via irrigation or DEN [21] (**Figure 2**). In DEN, an endoscope with one or two working ports is advanced through the previously placed, transluminal stent. Upon entering the WON, a number of tools, including forceps and snares are used to remove debris that would otherwise not be susceptible to removal with irrigation [21]. On average, 3–6 endoscopic interventions are necessary prior to resolution of necrosis [22].

DEN was first compared to surgical necrosectomy in the Pancreatitis, Endoscopic Transgastric vs. Primary Necrosectomy in Patients with Infected Necrosis (PENQUIN) Trial. In this trial, patients in the surgery group underwent a number of different operations, including 6 video-assisted retroperitoneal debridement (VARD) surgeries, 4 open necrosectomies, and 2 percutaneous drainage placements without need for more invasive therapy. The two patient who did not have a necrosectomy were excluded from final statistical analysis. All 10 patients in the endoscopic group had ultrasound guided stent placement, irrigation, and DEN. Following intervention, the rates of new-onset organ failure and pancreatic fistula were lower in the endoscopic group. The trial also compared the groups with regard to a composite clinical outcome, which included major post-operative complications and mortality, and found a lower rate in the endoscopic group [23, 24]. These findings were later replicated in the Minimally-invasive Surgery Versus Endoscopy Randomized (MISER) Trial. Additionally, MISER showed lower rates of pancreatic fistula formation and a higher quality of life at 3 months after surgery in the endoscopic group [25]. In the Transluminal Endoscopic Step-up Approach Versus Minimally-invasive Surgical Step-up Approach in Patients with Infected Necrotizing Pancreatitis (TENSION) Trial, a larger randomized trial, no difference in mortality was observed. However, the rates of pancreatic fistula and length of stay favored the endoscopic group [26].

Percutaneous drainage is preferable in patients that are deemed too unstable to tolerate endoscopic drainage or if the area of necrosis extends into a dependent

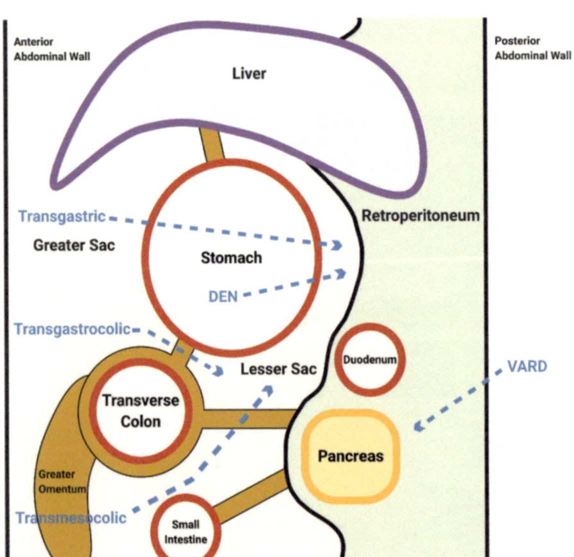

Figure 2.
Surgical approaches to Necrosectomy. Access the lesser sac and retroperitoneum for the purposes of pancreatic necrosectomy can be achieve through a number of approaches. Direct endoscopic necrosectomy (DEN) is performed by accessing the stomach via the esophagus and then creating a posterior gastrotomy. The transgastric approach, performed laparoscopically or open, requires both an anterior and a posterior gastrotomy. The lesser sac can also be accessed by opening the gastrocolic ligament or transverse mesocolon, either by traversing a previously established, drainage tract or with a surgical approach.

space, such as the paracolic gutters or pelvis. It is also an acceptable alternative when endoscopic drainage is unavailable or not technically feasible, specifically in the setting of ANC, when there is no capsule that could support an endoscopic stent [27].

Percutaneous drainage is usually CT-guided, although ultrasound-guided drainage can also be performed. These drains may be transperitoneal, with the external portion of the drain fixed in the anterior abdominal wall. These drains may also be placed through the flank, directly into the retroperitoneum, without traversing the peritoneum. In addition to draining ANC and WON, percutaneous drains can also be used for irrigation [28].

Although percutaneous drainage is successful as monotherapy in some patients, patients with larger areas of necrosis, multifocal necrosis, incomplete liquefaction, and pre-procedural organ failure are less likely to be adequately treated. While some of these factors can be overcome with larger drainage catheters, for these reasons, percutaneous drainage remains a bridge to therapy, allowing patients to survive the acute period of disease, and undergo definitive management later, with improved outcomes [26, 29, 30].

4. General considerations for surgical management

Surgical management may be minimally-invasive or open, but has the same two primary goals: obtaining source control by removing as much necrotic tissue as possible and providing access for irrigation and drainage. As a general principle, minimally-invasive approaches are preferred to open necrosectomy as first-line treatment. The improved outcomes of minimally-invasive technique lead to development of the "step-up" approach to management, which begins with percutaneous or endoscopic intervention, followed by a progression to surgical intervention as indicated by unresolved disease. However, the final treatment decision is dictated by the patient, surgeon, and available resources. A second principle is that surgical intervention should be delayed as long as possible in order to improve outcomes. Operating during the early, acute phase of pancreatitis, especially in the presence of ANC, rather than WON, is associated with higher morbidity and mortality regardless of surgical approach. A third principle is that long-term nutritional access, through a gastrostomy or gastrojejunostomy tube, should be obtained prior to concluding the procedure if no other method for enteral feeding has been established. Fourth, a cholecystectomy may also be performed if gallstones were implicated in the etiology of pancreatitis, provided the patient is adequately stable to undergo an additional procedure (**Figure 1**).

5. Minimally-invasive necrosectomy

VARD is a technique, used as the final phase of the step-up approach, where the retroperitoneum is accessed through a previously established, left flank, percutaneous drainage tract (**Figure 2**). The tract is then serially dilated, in order to accommodate progressively larger drainage catheters. At the time of surgery, in order to facilitate introduction of laparoscopic instruments, a small, 4–6 centimeter incision is made where the tract exits the skin. After confirming entry into the WON with a probe, tissue and fluid are removed with suction. The laparoscope is then inserted, with or without CO_2 insufflation, for continued debridement under direct visualization, using blunt laparoscopic forceps. Following debridement, again under direct visualization, large drainage catheters or chest tubes, 28-French or greater, are placed. After surgery, these catheters are used for repeated lavage as well as for drainage [31].

The superiority of VARD, and the step-up approach, compared to surgery for the treatment of necrotizing pancreatitis was first published in the Minimally-invasive Step-up Approach Versus Maximal Necrosectomy in Patients with Acute Necrotizing Pancreatitis (PANTER) Trial. In this study, 35% of the patients assigned to the step-up arm were successfully treated with percutaneous drainage alone. When comparing the step-up and surgical groups, the step-up group was less likely to have new-onset organ failure, less likely to develop an incisional hernia, and had an overall lower rate of endocrine insufficiency. However, the mortality rate was not significantly different, 19% in the step-up group versus 16% in surgery group [31].

A similar procedure, percutaneous endoscopic necrosectomy (PEN), can be performed utilizing a previously established percutaneous drainage tract. Unlike VARD, PEN utilizes a flexible endoscope, as compared to a rigid laparoscope. Because the endoscope has working ports, in addition to irrigation and suction, an additional incision around the tract is not needed. Also unlike VARD, PEN can be performed at bedside, with conscious sedation [32].

PEN was shown to be effective in a large, prospective study of 171 patients with infected pancreatic necrosis. The primary outcome investigated was control of sepsis and resolution of the infected collection. In this study, 18 of 26 (69%) patients with infected ANC and 23 of 27 (85%) with infected WON who underwent PEN were successfully treated, while the remainder required surgical necrosectomy. Predictors of failure included >50% parenchymal necrosis and early organ failure. ANC was not predictive. The overall mortality rate for this study was 38% [32, 33]. Although this technique has not been directly compared to surgery, VARD, or transmural endoscopy, this study demonstrated the safety and utility of PEN in patients with infected pancreatic necrosis.

Regardless of the type of minimally-invasive drainage, VARD or PEN, it has been shown that the "step-up approach," beginning with drainage and progressing to debridement, is superior to upfront surgical approaches in terms of mortality, rates of pancreaticocutaneous fistula formation, and long-term morbidity [25, 30, 34].

6. Transgastric necrosectomy

In addition to utilizing a percutaneous drainage tract for necrosectomy, access can also be gained through the stomach. By entering the abdomen and opening the anterior wall of the stomach and then opening the posterior aspect of the stomach, access to the lesser sac and underlying pancreas is achieved (**Figure 2**). An aperture between the WON and posterior wall of the stomach is then created, either with sutures or by stapling, providing a definitive drainage tract. This tract is then used for necrosectomy following the same principles as DEN.

This approach is most well suited for WON limited to the lesser sac. When there is extensive necrosis extending to the retroperitoneum or paracolic gutters, VARD or traditional necrosectomy are more appropriate, due to the limited exposure with this method. These limitations are counterbalanced by the minimal amount of mobilization required to enter the lesser sac by the transgastric method [35].

When performed laparoscopically, five ports are typically placed; in addition to an umbilical port, two ports are placed in the right upper quadrant, one port is placed in the left upper quadrant, and one port in the epigastrium. After entering the abdomen and creating the anterior gastrotomy, an ultrasound is used to identify the necrosis and plan the locations of the posterior gastrotomy. Ultrasound is adjunctive to preoperative imaging, which is also essential to surgical planning.

Both anterior and posterior gastrotomies should be made after placement of stay sutures. Upon entering the lesser sac, necrosectomy should be performed with blunt instruments, such as a ring forceps, taking great care to remove only loose material and avoid avulsing adherent tissue or vessels that may be bridging the area of necrosis. Following necrosectomy, a cystogastrostomy is created with an endoscopic stapler, or suture. The anterior gastrotomy is then closed with sutures or with a stapler [36].

When performed open, an upper midline incision is made, and the procedure proceeds in the same fashion as in the laparoscopic procedure. One difference in the open procedure is that many surgeons elect to use digital dissection for the necrosectomy, as opposed to instruments [37].

Open and laparoscopic approaches to transgastric drainage have been shown to have similar outcomes. In a recent retrospective review of patients from three tertiary referral centers, rates of morbidity, including rates of reoperation and hemorrhage, and mortality were not significantly different. However, the patients who underwent laparoscopic drainage had a higher rate of readmission. It should be noted that the overall mortality in this study was 2% at an average follow-up of 21 months, significantly less than reported elsewhere in the literature. The overall morbidity rate of 38% is in alignment with commonly reported rates elsewhere in literature [38].

Although surgical transgastric necrosectomy is relatively well tolerated, outcomes favor endoscopic transgastric drainage. Meta-analysis comparing the two show lower rates of overall major complications, pancreatic fistula formation, post-procedural organ failure, and hernia with an endoscopic approach. However, the overall rate of clinical resolution, post-operative bleeding, endocrine dysfunction, exocrine insufficiency, and mortality were not significantly different [39]. Thus, surgical transgastric necrosectomy is a valid alternative to other approaches of necrosectomy in the absence of an experienced endoscopist or at a center without access to advanced endoscopic tools.

7. Laparoscopic and open necrosectomy

Although utilization of a drainage tract and the transgastric approach are important for management of pancreatic necrosis, traditional laparoscopic and open necrosectomy methods also continue to be utilized.

For laparoscopic necrosectomy, patients are typically placed in lithotomy position, with the operating surgeon standing between the legs. An umbilical port is placed first. Upon entering the abdomen, a diagnostic laparoscopy should be performed. Subsequently, two left lateral ports and an epigastric port are placed. In some cases, a hand-assist port is placed to augment dissection and removal of tissue. Following lysis of adhesions, a transgastrocolic, for pancreatic head or body necrosis, or transmesocolic, for pancreatic tail necrosis, approach to retrogastric necrosectomy can be taken (**Figure 2**). Upon entering the area of necrosis, blunt instruments are used to remove loose, necrotic tissue. This tissue is then placed into an endocatch bag for removal from the abdomen. Dissection is alternated with irrigation and suction to remove as much necrotic tissue as possible [40]. Once the necrosectomy is complete, large drainage catheters are placed in the cavity, which also allow for post-operative irrigation. At this time, consideration should also be given to cholecystectomy, if gallstones were implicated in the development of pancreatitis, and to nutritional access. Depending on the specific study, mortality for patients who require laparoscopic necrosectomy ranges from 10 to 18%. Rates of reoperation also vary widely, ranging from 11 to 38% [41, 42].

The most invasive procedure used for the treatment of pancreatic necrosis is the open debridement. This technique is reserved for patients that fail other less invasive techniques, or patients who require concurrent intervention for another intraabdominal process, such as bowel ischemia or abdominal compartment syndrome. Unless midline laparotomy is required for another indication, the abdomen can be opened with bilateral, subcostal incisions. The gastrocolic ligament is then opened, and the stomach is reflected superiorly, exposing the lesser sac (**Figure 2**). The transverse mesocolon is then opened, exposing the retroperitoneum. The hepatic and splenic flexures of the transverse colon are often taken down at this point. A Kocher maneuver may also be necessary if the area of necrosis involves the head of the pancreas. Once the pancreas is adequately exposed, blunt debridement can begin. This is usually accomplished with digital dissection or with lavage in order to minimize the risk of bleeding or bile duct injury. These risks must be balances with adequate removal of loose, nonviable tissue. Wide drainage of the area with a sumping tube (i.e. Abramson drain) can facilitate continue lavage and debridement. The quality of the initial necrosectomy predicts the need for subsequent operations.

After necrosectomy, the abdomen may be kept open, with packing in place, to allow for repeated removal of necrotic tissue. Alternatively, the closed packing technique can also be used. This technique consists of filling the cavity created by the necrosectomy with gauze-filled Penrose drains. The drains are removed one at a time, until the cavity closes [43]. A third option is continuous irrigation, where large catheters are placed into the lesser sac under direct visualization. Additional drainage catheters are left in the peritoneal cavity. The abdomen is then closed and the large catheters are used for continuous installation of hypertonic fluid [44].

As in patients who undergo laparoscopic necrosectomy, the rates of morbidity and mortality following open necrosectomy are high. Rates of post-operative morbidity range from 34 to 95% and mortality ranges from 6 to 47%, depending on the pre-operative severity of illness. Rates of reoperation vary depending on the packing technique. When the abdomen is left open, reoperation is planned rather than required because of deterioration or other complications, such as hemorrhage. Depending on the study, when the abdomen is left open, patients may return to the operating room from 1 to 17 time. Comparatively, relaparotomy is required in 17% of patients treated with closed packing require and 17–27% of patients treated with continuous irrigation. Rates of pancreatic fistula also differ depending on packing technique with a 25–46% rate in open abdomens, 53% rate in closed packing, and 13–19% rate with continuous irrigation [45].

The outcomes for both of these techniques are improved when intervention can be delayed at least 3 weeks. Delayed necrosectomy is associated with lower rates of exocrine and endocrine insufficiency, adverse post-operative events, including bleeding, and mortality [17, 46]. Early surgical intervention only provides a survival benefit in the case of decompression of abdominal compartment syndrome [47, 48].

When compared directly, in a retrospective case series, the rates of pancreatic fistula, post-operative pulmonary infections, and surgical site infections were all significantly lower with laparoscopic necrosectomy. Additionally, patients who underwent laparoscopic necrosectomy also had a shorter length of stay, but a longer initial operation. There was no difference in need for reoperation, overall morbidity, or mortality. It should be noted that mortality was very low compared to other literature in this study, 5.9% in the open group and 4% in the laparoscopic group [49].

8. Disconnected pancreatic duct syndrome

While parenchymal destruction in pancreatic necrosis confers significant morbidity and mortality, the seriousness of this condition can be further compounded by concurrent disruption of the pancreatic duct. Disconnected pancreatic duct syndrome (DPDS) occurs when the remnant of pancreas distal to the necrosis, and duct disruption, remains viable and continues to release digestive enzymes into the retroperitoneum. DPDS most commonly occurs in the setting of severe acute pancreatitis, and can be found in up to 46% of patients with pancreatic necrosis [50]. DPDS can also occur as the result of trauma and chronic pancreatitis. The clinical presentation of DPDS is heterogenous. Some patients are asymptomatic and the injury is incidentally diagnosed on radiology. While others may have early satiety due to the size of the resulting fluid collection or symptomatic ascites [51, 52].

DPDS is an often overlooked complication due to the low accuracy of imaging in differentiating between full-thickness pancreatic necrosis, affecting the pancreatic duct, and partial thickness or peripancreatic necrosis. Often multiple imaging modalities are required for accurate diagnosis, which in turn leads to delays in diagnosis, increased morbidity, and increased costs [53–55]. Diagnostic criteria for DPDS include: necrosis of ≥2 cm of pancreatic parenchyma, viable pancreatic tissue distal to the area of necrosis, and extravasation of contrast when injected into the main pancreatic duct during ERCP [56].

Once DPDS is diagnosed, choice of intervention is dependent on the patient's clinical condition and the phase of disease. As in pancreatic necrosis without DPDS, intervention during the acute phase, when inflammation is high, is not only challenging, but also hazardous. Although the historical standard of care for these patients was surgery, if a patient deteriorates during the acute phase, initial therapy should be percutaneous or endoscopic. Percutaneous drainage, although useful as a temporizing measure, especially in unstable patients, is unlikely to succeed as monotherapy [57, 58]. Although success rates are dependent on the extent of necrosis, transpapillary and transmural endoscopic interventions have better short-term outcomes, with up to an 87% success rate of fistula resolution [50, 59, 60]. However, in order for endoscopic treatment to be successful, multiple interventions are often required, including hybrid approaches with percutaneous drains. Further, long-term data regarding patency and migration of indwelling stents is not available [60, 61]. Thus, percutaneous and endoscopic treatments remain temporizing measures, rather than definitive treatment, for DPDS, except for in patients who are poor surgical candidates [62].

Once a patient reaches the late stage of disease, or if a patient deteriorates despite optimal percutaneous and endoscopic intervention during the acute phase, surgery becomes the primary treatment for DPDS. Because of the technical difficulty of operating in the retroperitoneum after tissue planes have been obscured by inflammation, and because of the frequency of splenic vein thrombosis, and resulting sinistral portal hypertension, this operation is usually performed with a midline laparotomy and not laparoscopically [63].

Surgery for DPDS consists of resection of the distal, disconnected pancreas, and creation of internal drainage tracts. These techniques may be used independently or in combination. When the entirety of the disconnected pancreas is resected, splenectomy is also performed in almost all cases. However, when a pancreatojejunostomy, pancreaticogastrostomy, or fistuloenterostomy is made with the viable distal pancreas, the spleen may be preserved, in addition to preserving the pancreatic remnant. In this way, internal drainage not only provide a conduit for pancreatic secretions, but also decreases the risk of exocrine pancreatic insufficiency and diabetes. Importantly, patients who undergo internal drainage, compared to other surgical modalities, also have lower incidence of organ failure, development of pancreatic fistula, and need for long-term percutaneous drainage [50, 64].

9. Conclusions

Pancreatic necrosis is a significant and challenging disease process with mortality reaching beyond 30% in most studies. Intervention begins with supportive care and nutritional support. However, invasive therapy is often needed, especially when necrosis becomes infected.

First-line interventions for pancreatic necrosis may be percutaneous or transmural endoscopic drainage depending on if the necrosis is encapsulated, the accessibility of the necrosis, the patient's clinical condition, and the capabilities of the hospital. These minimally-invasive interventions are often successful as monotherapy, without the need for further intervention. They are also preferable to open or laparoscopic necrosectomy when performed as part of a step-up approach.

Despite all of the improvement in minimally-invasive management of pancreatic necrosis, some percentage of patients continue to require surgical intervention. Both laparoscopic and open approaches have been shown to be effective via transgastric, transgastrocolic, and transmesocolic routes.

When pancreatic necrosis is further complicated by a disconnected pancreatic duct, although minimally-invasive management has been described and shown to be effective, surgical management remains standard of care.

Despite the advances in care driven by clinical trials and new technology, management of pancreatic necrosis remains difficult. Further study is needed to reduce the morbidity and mortality of this devastating disease.

Acknowledgements

All authors contributed equally to the authorship of this chapter.

Conflict of interest

The authors declare no conflicts of interest.

Notes/thanks/other declarations

The authors would like to thank the leadership of the Department of Surgery at the Donald and Barbara School of Medicine at Hofstra/Northwell, including Drs. Vihas Patel and Gene Coppa, for sponsoring the writing of this chapter.

Appendices and nomenclature

ACN	acute necrotic collection
CT	computed tomography
DEN	direct endoscopic necrosectomy
DPDS	disconnected pancreatic duct syndrome
ERCP	endoscopic retrograde cholangiopancreatography

EUS	endoscopic ultrasound
FNA	fine needle aspiration
HU	Hounsfield units
PEN	percutaneous endoscopic necrosectomy
SEMS	self-expanding metal stent
TPN	total parenteral nutrition
WON	walled of necrosis
VARD	video-assisted retroperitoneal debridement

Author details

Dane Thompson[1,2,3,4], Siavash Bolourani[1,2,3,4] and Matthew Giangola[4*]

1 The Feinstein Institutes for Medical Research, Manhasset, New York, United States

2 Elmezzi Graduate School of Molecular Medicine, Manhasset, New York, United States

3 Donald and Barbara Zucker School of Medicine at Hofstra/Northwell, Manhasset, New York, United States

4 Department of Surgery, Donald and Barbara Zucker School of Medicine at Hofstra Northwell School of Medicine, Manhasset, New York, United States

*Address all correspondence to: mgiangola@northwell.edu

References

[1] Banks PA, Bollen TL, Dervenis C, Gooszen HG, Johnson CD, Sarr MG, et al. Classification of acute pancreatitis—2012: revision of the Atlanta classification and definitions by international consensus. Gut 2013;62:102-111. https://doi.org/10.1136/gutjnl-2012-302779.

[2] Kokosis G, Perez A, Pappas TN. Surgical management of necrotizing pancreatitis: an overview. World J Gastroenterol 2014;20:16106-12. https://doi.org/10.3748/wjg.v20.i43.16106.

[3] Türkvatan A, Erden A, Türkoğlu MA, Seçil M, Yener Ö. Imaging of acute pancreatitis and its complications. Part 1: Acute pancreatitis. Diagn Interv Imaging 2015;96:151-60. https://doi.org/10.1016/j.diii.2013.12.017.

[4] Koo BC, Chinogureyi A, Shaw AS. Imaging acute pancreatitis. Br J Radiol 2010;83:104-12. https://doi.org/10.1259/bjr/13359269.

[5] Petrov MS, Kukosh MV, Emelyanov NV. A randomized controlled trial of enteral versus parenteral feeding in patients with predicted severe acute pancreatitis shows a significant reduction in mortality and in infected pancreatic complications with total enteral nutrition. Dig Surg 2006;23:336-44; discussion 344-345. https://doi.org/10.1159/000097949.

[6] Wu X-M, Ji K-Q, Wang H-Y, Li G-F, Zang B, Chen W-M. Total enteral nutrition in prevention of pancreatic necrotic infection in severe acute pancreatitis. Pancreas 2010;39:248-51. https://doi.org/10.1097/MPA.0b013e3181bd6370.

[7] Wu X-M, Liao Y-W, Wang H-Y, Ji K-Q, Li G-F, Zang B. When to initialize enteral nutrition in patients with severe acute pancreatitis? A retrospective review in a single institution experience (2003-2013). Pancreas 2015;44:507-11. https://doi.org/10.1097/MPA.0000000000000293.

[8] Leppäniemi A, Tolonen M, Tarasconi A, Segovia-Lohse H, Gamberini E, Kirkpatrick AW, et al. 2019 WSES guidelines for the management of severe acute pancreatitis. World J Emerg Surg 2019;14:27. https://doi.org/10.1186/s13017-019-0247-0.

[9] Jj H, N S, A S, As R, Ss I, Si G, et al. Outcomes of Infected versus Symptomatic Sterile Walled-Off Pancreatic Necrosis Treated with a Minimally Invasive Therapy. Gut Liver 2019;13. https://doi.org/10.5009/gnl18234.

[10] Beger HG, Rau BM. Severe acute pancreatitis: Clinical course and management. World J Gastroenterol WJG 2007;13:5043. https://doi.org/10.3748/wjg.v13.i38.5043.

[11] Schepers NJ, Bakker OJ, Besselink MG, Ali UA, Bollen TL, Gooszen HG, et al. Impact of characteristics of organ failure and infected necrosis on mortality in necrotising pancreatitis. Gut 2019;68:1044-51. https://doi.org/10.1136/gutjnl-2017-314657.

[12] Choe KA. Imaging in pancreatic infection. J Hepatobiliary Pancreat Surg 2003;10:401-5. https://doi.org/10.1007/s00534-002-0713-y.

[13] Baron TH, DiMaio CJ, Wang AY, Morgan KA. American Gastroenterological Association Clinical Practice Update: Management of Pancreatic Necrosis. Gastroenterology 2020;158:67-75.e1. https://doi.org/10.1053/j.gastro.2019.07.064.

[14] Isenmann R, Rünzi M, Kron M, Kahl S, Kraus D, Jung N, et al. Prophylactic antibiotic treatment in patients with predicted severe acute pancreatitis: a placebo-controlled, double-blind trial. Gastroenterology 2004;126:997-1004. https://doi.org/10.1053/j.gastro.2003.12.050.

[15] Dellinger EP, Tellado JM, Soto NE, Ashley SW, Barie PS, Dugernier T, et al. Early antibiotic treatment for severe acute necrotizing pancreatitis: a randomized, double-blind, placebo-controlled study. Ann Surg 2007;245:674-83. https://doi.org/10.1097/01.sla.0000250414.09255.84.

[16] García-Barrasa A, Borobia FG, Pallares R, Jorba R, Poves I, Busquets J, et al. A double-blind, placebo-controlled trial of ciprofloxacin prophylaxis in patients with acute necrotizing pancreatitis. J Gastrointest Surg Off J Soc Surg Aliment Tract 2009;13:768-74. https://doi.org/10.1007/s11605-008-0773-7.

[17] Bugiantella W, Rondelli F, Boni M, Stella P, Polistena A, Sanguinetti A, et al. Necrotizing pancreatitis: A review of the interventions. Int J Surg 2016;28:S163-71. https://doi.org/10.1016/j.ijsu.2015.12.038.

[18] van Brunschot S, Fockens P, Bakker OJ, Besselink MG, Voermans RP, Poley J-W, et al. Endoscopic transluminal necrosectomy in necrotising pancreatitis: a systematic review. Surg Endosc 2014;28:1425-38. https://doi.org/10.1007/s00464-013-3382-9.

[19] van Baal MC, van Santvoort HC, Bollen TL, Bakker OJ, Besselink MG, Gooszen HG, et al. Systematic review of percutaneous catheter drainage as primary treatment for necrotizing pancreatitis. Br J Surg 2011;98:18-27. https://doi.org/10.1002/bjs.7304.

[20] Patel R, Gardner TB. Early versus late necrotic pancreatic fluid collection drainage: Does timing make a difference? Gastrointest Endosc 2020;91:1310-1. https://doi.org/10.1016/j.gie.2020.02.023.

[21] Kumar N, Conwell DL, Thompson CC. Direct Endoscopic Necrosectomy Versus Step-Up Approach for Walled-Off Pancreatic Necrosis: Comparison of Clinical Outcome and Health Care Utilization. Pancreas 2014;43:1334-1339. https://doi.org/10.1097/MPA.0000000000000213.

[22] Jha AK, Goenka MK, Kumar R, Suchismita A. Endotherapy for pancreatic necrosis: An update. JGH Open 2019;3:80-8. https://doi.org/10.1002/jgh3.12109.

[23] Bakker OJ, van Santvoort HC, van Brunschot S, Geskus RB, Besselink MG, Bollen TL, et al. Endoscopic Transgastric vs Surgical Necrosectomy for Infected Necrotizing Pancreatitis: A Randomized Trial. JAMA 2012;307:1053. https://doi.org/10.1001/jama.2012.276.

[24] Hines OJ, Donald GW. Endoscopic Transgastric Necrosectomy for Infected Necrotizing Pancreatitis. JAMA J Am Med Assoc 2012;307:1084-5. https://doi.org/10.1001/jama.2012.306.

[25] Bang JY, Arnoletti JP, Holt BA, Sutton B, Hasan MK, Navaneethan U, et al. An Endoscopic Transluminal Approach, Compared With Minimally Invasive Surgery, Reduces Complications and Costs for Patients With Necrotizing Pancreatitis. Gastroenterology 2019;156:1027-1040.e3. https://doi.org/10.1053/j.gastro.2018.11.031.

[26] van Brunschot S, van Grinsven J, van Santvoort HC, Bakker OJ, Besselink MG, Boermeester MA, et al. Endoscopic or surgical step-up approach for infected necrotising pancreatitis: a multicentre

randomised trial. The Lancet 2018;391:51-8. https://doi.org/10.1016/S0140-6736(17)32404-2.

[27] Sharma P. CT Guided Percutaneous Drainage in Necrotizing Pancreatitis – Highly Successful In Appropriately Selected Patients - Single Center Experience 2019:6.

[28] Tyberg A, Karia K, Gabr M, Desai A, Doshi R, Gaidhane M, et al. Management of pancreatic fluid collections: A comprehensive review of the literature. World J Gastroenterol 2016;22:2256-70. https://doi.org/10.3748/wjg.v22.i7.2256.

[29] Wroński M, Cebulski W, Karkocha D, Słodkowski M, Wysocki Ł, Jankowski M, et al. Ultrasound-guided percutaneous drainage of infected pancreatic necrosis. Surg Endosc 2013;27:2841-8. https://doi.org/10.1007/s00464-013-2831-9.

[30] van Santvoort HC, Besselink MG, Bakker OJ, Hofker HS, Boermeester MA, Dejong CH, et al. A Step-up Approach or Open Necrosectomy for Necrotizing Pancreatitis. N Engl J Med 2010;362:1491-502. https://doi.org/10.1056/NEJMoa0908821.

[31] van Santvoort HC, Besselink MGH, Horvath KD, Sinanan MN, Bollen TL, van Ramshorst B, et al. Videoscopic assisted retroperitoneal debridement in infected necrotizing pancreatitis. HPB 2007;9:156-9. https://doi.org/10.1080/13651820701225688.

[32] Jain S, Padhan R, Bopanna S, Jain SK, Dhingra R, Dash NR, et al. Percutaneous Endoscopic Step-Up Therapy Is an Effective Minimally Invasive Approach for Infected Necrotizing Pancreatitis. Dig Dis Sci 2020;65:615-22. https://doi.org/10.1007/s10620-019-05696-2.

[33] Trikudanathan G. Percutaneous Endoscopic Necrosectomy (PEN): Is the PEN Mightier Than the VARD? Dig Dis Sci 2020;65:339-41. https://doi.org/10.1007/s10620-019-05790-5.

[34] Hollemans RA, Bakker OJ, Boermeester MA, Bollen TL, Bosscha K, Bruno MJ, et al. Superiority of Step-up Approach vs Open Necrosectomy in Long-term Follow-up of Patients With Necrotizing Pancreatitis. Gastroenterology 2019;156:1016-26. https://doi.org/10.1053/j.gastro.2018.10.045.

[35] Zyromski NJ, Nakeeb A, House MG, Jester AL. Transgastric Pancreatic Necrosectomy: How I Do It. J Gastrointest Surg Off J Soc Surg Aliment Tract 2016;20:445-9. https://doi.org/10.1007/s11605-015-3058-y.

[36] Kulkarni S, Bogart A, Buxbaum J, Matsuoka L, Selby R, Parekh D. Surgical transgastric debridement of walled off pancreatic necrosis: an option for patients with necrotizing pancreatitis. Surg Endosc 2015;29:575-82. https://doi.org/10.1007/s00464-014-3700-x.

[37] Sasnur P, Nidoni R, Baloorkar R, Sindgikar V, Shankar B. Extended Open Transgastric Necrosectomy (EOTN) as a Safer Procedure for Necrotizing Pancreatitis. J Clin Diagn Res JCDR 2014;8:NR01-02. https://doi.org/10.7860/JCDR/2013/8196.4600.

[38] Driedger M, Zyromski NJ, Visser BC, Jester A, Sutherland FR, Nakeeb A, et al. Surgical Transgastric Necrosectomy for Necrotizing Pancreatitis: A Single-stage Procedure for Walled-off Pancreatic Necrosis. Ann Surg 2020;271:163-8. https://doi.org/10.1097/SLA.0000000000003048.

[39] Luo D, Liu X, Du J, Liu J, Chen X, Zhou P, et al. Endoscopic Transgastric Versus Surgical Approach for Infected Necrotizing Pancreatitis: A Systematic Review and Meta-Analysis. Surg Laparosc Endosc Percutan Tech

2019;29:141-9. https://doi.org/10.1097/SLE.0000000000000632.

[40] Mathew MJ, Parmar AK, Sahu D, Reddy PK. Laparoscopic necrosectomy in acute necrotizing pancreatitis: Our experience. J Minimal Access Surg 2014;10:126-31. https://doi.org/10.4103/0972-9941.134875.

[41] Parekh D. Laparoscopic-assisted pancreatic necrosectomy: A new surgical option for treatment of severe necrotizing pancreatitis. Arch Surg Chic Ill 1960 2006;141:895-902; discussion 902-903. https://doi.org/10.1001/archsurg.141.9.895.

[42] Gagner null. Laparoscopic Treatment of Acute Necrotizing Pancreatitis. Semin Laparosc Surg 1996;3:21-8. https://doi.org/10.1053/SLAS00300021.

[43] Rodriguez JR, Razo AO, Targarona J, Thayer SP, Rattner DW, Warshaw AL, et al. Debridement and Closed Packing for Sterile or Infected Necrotizing Pancreatitis. Ann Surg 2008;247:294-9. https://doi.org/10.1097/SLA.0b013e31815b6976.

[44] Rau B, Bothe A, Beger HG. Surgical treatment of necrotizing pancreatitis by necrosectomy and closed lavage: changing patient characteristics and outcome in a 19-year, single-center series. Surgery 2005;138:28-39. https://doi.org/10.1016/j.surg.2005.03.010.

[45] Werner J, Feuerbach S, Uhl W, Büchler MW. Management of acute pancreatitis: from surgery to interventional intensive care. Gut 2005;54:426-36. https://doi.org/10.1136/gut.2003.035907.

[46] Mier J, León EL, Castillo A, Robledo F, Blanco R. Early versus late necrosectomy in severe necrotizing pancreatitis. Am J Surg 1997;173:71-5. https://doi.org/10.1016/S0002-9610(96)00425-4.

[47] Freeman ML, Werner J, Santvoort HCV, Baron TH, Besselink MG, Windsor JA, et al. Interventions for necrotizing pancreatitis: Summary of a multidisciplinary consensus conference. Pancreas 2012;41:1176-94. https://doi.org/10.1097/MPA.0b013e318269c660.

[48] Mentula P, Hienonen P, Kemppainen E, Puolakkainen P, Leppäniemi A. Surgical Decompression for Abdominal Compartment Syndrome in Severe Acute Pancreatitis. Arch Surg 2010;145:764-9. https://doi.org/10.1001/archsurg.2010.132.

[49] Tan J, Tan H, Hu B, Ke C, Ding X, Chen F, et al. Short-Term Outcomes from a Multicenter Retrospective Study in China Comparing Laparoscopic and Open Surgery for the Treatment of Infected Pancreatic Necrosis. J Laparoendosc Adv Surg Tech 2012;22:27-33. https://doi.org/10.1089/lap.2011.0248.

[50] Maatman TK, Roch AM, Lewellen KA, Heimberger MA, Ceppa EP, House MG, et al. Disconnected Pancreatic Duct Syndrome: Spectrum of Operative Management. J Surg Res 2020;247:297-303. https://doi.org/10.1016/j.jss.2019.09.068.

[51] Fischer TD, Gutman DS, Hughes SJ, Trevino JG, Behrns KE. Disconnected pancreatic duct syndrome: disease classification and management strategies. J Am Coll Surg 2014;219:704-12. https://doi.org/10.1016/j.jamcollsurg.2014.03.055.

[52] Rana SS, Sharma RK, Gupta R. Endoscopic management of pancreatic ascites due to duct disruption following acute necrotizing pancreatitis. JGH Open Open Access J Gastroenterol Hepatol 2019;3:111-6. https://doi.org/10.1002/jgh3.12113.

[53] Timmerhuis HC, van Dijk SM, Verdonk RC, Bollen TL, Bruno MJ,

Fockens P, et al. Various Modalities Accurate in Diagnosing a Disrupted or Disconnected Pancreatic Duct in Acute Pancreatitis: A Systematic Review. Dig Dis Sci 2020. https://doi.org/10.1007/s10620-020-06413-0.

[54] Chen Y, Jiang Y, Qian W, Yu Q, Dong Y, Zhu H, et al. Endoscopic transpapillary drainage in disconnected pancreatic duct syndrome after acute pancreatitis and trauma: long-term outcomes in 31 patients. BMC Gastroenterol 2019;19:54. https://doi.org/10.1186/s12876-019-0977-1.

[55] Verma S, Rana SS. Disconnected pancreatic duct syndrome: Updated review on clinical implications and management. Pancreatol Off J Int Assoc Pancreatol IAP Al 2020;20: 1035-44. https://doi.org/10.1016/j.pan.2020.07.402.

[56] Sandrasegaran K, Tann M, Jennings SG, Maglinte DD, Peter SD, Sherman S, et al. Disconnection of the pancreatic duct: an important but overlooked complication of severe acute pancreatitis. Radiogr Rev Publ Radiol Soc N Am Inc 2007;27:1389-400. https://doi.org/10.1148/rg.275065163.

[57] Nealon WH, Bhutani M, Riall TS, Raju G, Ozkan O, Neilan R. A unifying concept: pancreatic ductal anatomy both predicts and determines the major complications resulting from pancreatitis. J Am Coll Surg 2009;208:790-9; discussion 799-801. https://doi.org/10.1016/j.jamcollsurg.2008.12.027.

[58] Larsen M, Kozarek RA. Management of Disconnected Pancreatic Duct Syndrome. Curr Treat Options Gastroenterol 2016;14:348-59. https://doi.org/10.1007/s11938-016-0098-7.

[59] Irani S, Gluck M, Ross A, Gan SI, Crane R, Brandabur JJ, et al. Resolving external pancreatic fistulas in patients with disconnected pancreatic duct syndrome: using rendezvous techniques to avoid surgery (with video). Gastrointest Endosc 2012;76:586-593.e1-3. https://doi.org/10.1016/j.gie.2012.05.006.

[60] Varadarajulu S, Noone TC, Tutuian R, Hawes RH, Cotton PB. Predictors of outcome in pancreatic duct disruption managed by endoscopic transpapillary stent placement. Gastrointest Endosc 2005;61:568-75. https://doi.org/10.1016/s0016-5107(04)02832-9.

[61] Bang JY, Wilcox CM, Navaneethan U, Hasan MK, Peter S, Christein J, et al. Impact of Disconnected Pancreatic Duct Syndrome on the Endoscopic Management of Pancreatic Fluid Collections. Ann Surg 2018;267: 561-8. https://doi.org/10.1097/SLA.0000000000002082.

[62] Nadkarni NA, Kotwal V, Sarr MG, Swaroop Vege S. Disconnected Pancreatic Duct Syndrome: Endoscopic Stent or Surgeon's Knife? Pancreas 2015;44:16-22. https://doi.org/10.1097/MPA.0000000000000216.

[63] Howard TJ, Moore SA, Saxena R, Matthews DE, Schmidt CM, Wiebke EA. Pancreatic duct strictures are a common cause of recurrent pancreatitis after successful management of pancreatic necrosis. Surgery 2004;136:909-16. https://doi.org/10.1016/j.surg.2004.06.028.

[64] van Dijk SM, Timmerhuis HC, Verdonk RC, Reijnders E, Bruno MJ, Fockens P, et al. Treatment of disrupted and disconnected pancreatic duct in necrotizing pancreatitis: A systematic review and meta-analysis. Pancreatol Off J Int Assoc Pancreatol IAP Al 2019;19:905-15. https://doi.org/10.1016/j.pan.2019.08.006.

Chapter 6

Current Approaches in Chronic Pancreatitis

Didem Saka, Can Boynukara, Elif Reyyan Çadırcıbaşı and Gürhan Şişman

Abstract

Chronic pancreatitis is a fibroinflammatory syndrome of the pancreas that results in exocrine and endocrine pancreatic insufficiency and chronic pain. It can be seen in all age groups depending on the etiologic factors. It is believed that alcohol is one of the major etiologic factors of chronic pancreatitis, but it is now recognized that alcohol is responsible for 50% of the cases. Mutations in many genes such as PRSS1, SPINK1, CTRC, CFTR are identified as causative or predisposing factors for CP. Early diagnosis and staging of CP are still a challenge in clinic. Although the chief complaint of patients with CP is abdominal pain, CP can cause many disorders such as diabetes or metabolic bone diseases. The treatment of CP mainly depends on the severity of the disease and morphology of the pancreas. Medical therapy, endoscopy and surgery are all used for the treatment of CP and its complications.

Keywords: pancreas, chronic pancreatitis, endoscopy, gastroenterology, endosonography

1. Introduction

Chronic pancreatitis (CP) is characterized by fibroinflammatory inflammation of pancreatic tissue that causes progressive and irreversible destruction of the exocrine pancreas and loss of islets of Langerhans. The cause of the chronic pancreatitis is often multifactorial, involving chronic alcohol usage, recurrent acute pancreatitis attacks, structural or genetic anomalies.

2. Epidemiology

CP can be seen in all age groups depending on the etiologic factors. Although true prevalence is approximately < 50 per 100,000 adults, peaking in patients aged 46–55 years, the determination of its prevalence is difficult because of local standards and reporting bias. The incidence is predicted to be 4 to 5 new diagnoses per 100,000 yearly [1]. Data from Italian, Spanish, Chinese and Japanese surveys have the similar results as mentioned above [2].

CP is a slightly male predominant disease due to more alcohol and tobacco usage. Recently, several studies aimed to explain male sex predominance with the changes of the Claudin (CLDN)2 locus on the X chromosome in alcohol-induced chronic pancreatitis [3, 4].

Hospital admission for acute and chronic pancreatitis are increasing in the United States. Pancreatitis (acute and chronic) was among the three most common benign gastrointestinal diagnoses and accounted for a 12% increase in emergency room visits since 2006 according to US registry-based analysis that was published in 2019 [5]. Considering the stable or decreasing tobacco and alcohol use in most western countries and the probable unchanging prevalence of genetic risk factors, greater sensitivity of diagnostic testing can be the cause of increased hospital admissions. Approximately 3–35% of patients with a first episode of acute pancreatitis will progress to chronic pancreatitis over 3–8 years [6, 7]. Oppositely, only about 50% of patients with chronic pancreatitis had previously documented episodes of acute pancreatitis [8].

Black patients suffer more severe pain and disability and have more advanced morphological changes on the imaging techniques compared with white patients [9]. These results can be explained by more frequent usage of alcohol and tobacco in those patients. CP, like in many countries, is a male predominance disease in Turkey. The median age of the disease is 46 for male patients and 50 for female patients. The main etiological factor for the disease is alcohol abuse [10].

3. Etiology

It is believed that alcohol is one of the major etiologic factors of chronic pancreatitis, but it is now recognized that alcohol is responsible for 50% of the cases [3]. Therefore, stigmatization of patients with chronic pancreatitis as having an alcohol use disorder is often inaccurate and unfitting. It has been estimated that patients must consume 4–5 alcoholic drinks per day consistently for over 5 years to be at risk [11]. Alcohol exposure has several unwanted effects to the pancreas tissue. Despite common knowledge, it makes pancreas more susceptible to injury rather than directly causing chronic pancreatitis.

Usage of tobacco products is another risk factor for chronic pancreatitis. In the past, it was assumed cigarette smoking caused chronic pancreatitis due to concurrent alcohol consumption, but studies demonstrated a link between an independent and dose-dependent response of tobacco usage and chronic pancreatitis [12]. Also, cigarette smoking is a strong risk factor for recurrent acute pancreatitis which can eventually progress to chronic pancreatitis. Smoking is related to the induction of interleukin-22 secondary to aryl hydrocarbons, which promote pancreatic fibrosis [13].

Recurrent episodes of acute pancreatitis can lead to pancreatic fibrosis, gland atrophy, loss of islet of Langerhans which eventually progress into chronic pancreatitis.

Hereditary pancreatitis is another etiologic factor for developing chronic pancreatitis. It is observed as an autosomal dominant mutation of the cationic trypsinogen gene (PRSS1). Hereditary pancreatitis is an autosomal dominant disease with high penetrance up to 80% but some patients can also develop the PRSS1 gene mutation de novo.

Another mutation can also be the cause of chronic pancreatitis. Including genes that encode serine peptidase inhibitor Kazal type 1 (SPINK1), chymotrypsin C (CTRC), calcium-sensing receptor (CASR), claudin (CLDN2) and cystic fibrosis transmembrane conductance regulator (CFTR). Due to CFTR gene mutation cystic fibrosis is another etiologic risk factor for chronic pancreatitis. Also, Carboxypeptidase A1 (CPA1) and carboxyl ester lipase (CEL) gene mutations are thought to be increasing risk factors for chronic pancreatitis.

There are two unique subtypes of chronic pancreatitis. The first subtype is referred to as tropical pancreatitis (previously fibro calculous pancreatitis) which is mostly seen in Southeast Asia, especially in India. Previously, the cause of tropical pancreatitis was believed to be cassava root ingestion. However, this hypothesis has not been supported. Half of the patients who suffer from tropical pancreatitis show SPINK1 gene mutation, but the pathogenesis of the tropical pancreatitis remains unexplained [14].

The other subtype of chronic pancreatitis is autoimmune pancreatitis (AIP) which is subclassified as type 1 AIP (lymphoplasmacytic sclerosing pancreatitis) and type 2 AIP (idiopathic duct-centric pancreatitis). AIP, especially lymphoplasmacytic sclerosing pancreatitis is associated with IgG4-secreting plasma cells in the pancreas. Type 1 AIP has also extra pancreatic manifestations like sclerosing cholangitis and retroperitoneal fibrosis. Patients eventually develop pancreatic calcifications and pancreatic insufficiencies that are indistinguishable from chronic pancreatitis.

Less commonly, hypercalcemia (generally due to parathyroid adenoma), hypertriglyceridemia, autoimmune disorders (eg, celiac disease, inflammatory bowel diseases) can cause chronic pancreatitis.

Approximately 40% of the chronic pancreatitis patients' etiology is unknown [15].

4. Pathogenesis

The exact pathogenesis underlying the chronic pancreatitis is not totally defined. The disease most commonly occurs due to environmental factors such as alcohol and smoking or in patients with genetic abnormalities. However, idiopathic CP affects almost 50% of people with this condition [15]. Some hypotheses for the pathophysiology are proposed to explain the etiologic factors. These can give us ideas about the mechanism about the development of the chronic pancreatitis.

4.1 Toxic – metabolic

Excessive alcohol consumption is responsible for 50% of the chronic pancreatic cases [16]. Alcohol is also the best-known etiologic factor in the world, so that patients can be stigmatized with alcoholism and this leads to lower quality of life. It is shown that alcohol is toxic to acinar cells, pancreatic ducts and its microcirculation [17, 18]. It was supposed that alcohol causes to spasm of the sphincter of Oddi, and it affects the character of pancreatic fluid to favor the formation of protein plugs and stones, which eventually lead to chronic pancreatitis [19]. However, these two theories failed to fully explain the pathogenesis of the alcoholic pancreatitis, scientists focused on the acinar the effect of the alcohol on the acinar cells, which are full of thousands digestive enzyme molecules. Normally, the enzymes are produced as inactive precursors, packed into zymogen granules, and segregated from mainly lysosomal enzymes in order to avoid premature activation [19]. Alcohol leads to destabilization of lysosomes and zymogen granules via by oxidant stress produced by cholesteryl esters (CEs), which accumulate in the pancreas during ethanol consumption; and fatty acid ethyl esters (FAEEs), which are nonoxidative metabolites of alcohol. The enzyme synthesis is increased, but the secretion is also impaired. Therefore, it predisposes the gland to autodigestive injury. The cytokines released during prolonged injury and the ethanol itself via its metabolite acetaldehyde causes activation of the PSC (specific, highly plastic type of myofibroblast) leading to excess deposition of extra cellular matrix and active tissue remodeling and resulting in fibrosis and replacement of functional tissue [20–23]. Smoking is also common in patients with CP. It is convincingly demonstrated that smoking has an independent from alcohol, dose-dependent effect for developing CP. In addition, it is a facilitating factor for progressing of acute pancreatitis to CP. Furthermore, smoking promotes the fibrosis by inducing the IL-2 [13]. A potent toxic component of nicotine metabolite causes trypsinogen activation and cellular damage leading to pancreatitis [24].

4.2 Inappropriate protease activation

Pancreatic acinar cells secrete proteases as precursor enzymes, which are then activated by the serine protease in the duodenum [25]. Trypsin, the precursor of the major protease trypsinogen, starts the activation cascade of many other proteases, and itself in the duodenum (autoactivation). The natural inhibitors of the intrapancreatic activation are the SPINK1, trypsinogen degradation by CTRC and cathepsin L. Most genetic mutations associated with CP are trypsin dependent. Premature intrapancreatic activation or inappropriate inhibition of the trypsinogen can lead to pathologic event resulting in CP [26].

4.2.1 PRSS1 and PRSS2

Hereditary pancreatitis (HP) is a specific subtype of CP. The mutations in the human cationic trypsinogen (PRSS1) can cause the premature activation of the trypsinogen in various ways. 90% percent of the HP patients diagnosed with PRSS1 mutation carry one of the 3 mutations: p.N29I, p.R122C, or p.R122H in the heterozygous state. The p.N29I variant causes an increase in N-terminal processing, decreased CTRC -dependent degradation, and an increased propensity for autoactivation of the trypsin. The p.R122C and p.R122H mutations mainly prevent CTRC-mediated trypsinogen degradation [27–29].

There is no pathologic variants of human anionic trypsinogen (PRSS2) found in patients with CP. Even Genome wide association studies (GWASs) have identified a protective PRSS2 locus that slightly decreases CP risk, with a more pronounced effect in alcoholic [30].

4.2.2 SPINK1

The gene that encode serine peptidase inhibitor Kazal type 1 (SPINK1) is found to be associated with CP and commonly observed (40–50%) in tropical pancreatitis, which was referred as fibrocalculous pancreatitis [14]. The variant p.N34S in SPINK1 gene is ten times often in patient with CP compared to normal population [31]. However, the pathophysiologic mechanism is not yet known clearly although it is accepted as a major risk factor for CP.

4.2.3 CTRC

CTRC is a digestive protease synthesized and secreted by the pancreatic acinar cells as an inactive proenzyme (zymogen), which becomes activated in the duodenum. Physiologic functions include degradation of trypsin and trypsinogen, as an important defensive mechanism in chronic pancreatitis [32]. Besides, CTRC is not only a digestive enzyme but also plays a role in regulating the activity of other digestive enzymes such as stimulating autoactivation of human cationic trypsinogen [28]. Furthermore, CTRC is an essential co-activator of pro carboxypeptidase A1 (pro CPA1) and pro carboxypeptidase A2 (pro CPA2) [33].

Mutations in the *CTRC* gene have been shown to increase the risk of CP and they are 30% prevalent among patients with CP. The three main pathways explaining the increased risk of CP involve (i) impaired trypsinogen and/or trypsin degradation; (ii) impaired activation of A-type carboxypeptidases, and (iii) induction of ER stress due to defective secretion [32].

4.2.4 CTRB

CTRB1 and CTRB2 genes encode a member of the serine protease family of enzymes. The study by Rosendahl et al. reported the identification of *CTRB1-CTRB2* (chymotrypsin B1 and chymotrypsin B2) as a new chronic pancreatitis (CP) risk locus by means of GWAS. The inversion is found to decrease the CP risk by increasing trypsinogen degradation [34].

4.2.5 CELA3B

Recently, researchers found a new protease mutation linked to hereditary pancreatitis. The missense mutation in the gene encoding pancreas-specific protease elastase 3B (CELA3B), which upon secretion and activation by trypsin leads to uncontrolled proteolysis and recurrent pancreatitis [35].

4.3 Ductal dysfunction

After joining the common bile duct, the main pancreatic duct, after which both ducts perforate the medial side of the second portion of the duodenum. Therefore, any obstruction, compression or inflammation of the pancreatic tissue will increase the pressure within the pancreatic ducts leading to ductal dilation, stenosis and to atrophy of the acinar cells and replacement by fibrous tissue [36]. Long standing ductal obstructions by pseudocyst, calculi or pancreatic division can be a reason for recurrent pancreatitis attacks, which lead to eventually fibrosis and pancreatic insufficiency. Ductal obstruction can be also caused by concretions which increase the viscosity of the secretions and thereby promoting protein plugging [37].

A distinct form is the pancreatitis resulting due to a mutation in the cystic fibrosis transmembrane conductance regulator (CFTR) gene. CFTR is a chloride–bicarbonate channel expressed in the apical plasma membrane of secretory epithelia in many organs such as pancreas. The channel controls transepithelial fluid secretion and hence hydration of the epithelial luminal surfaces. It also controls the pH of the secretions, which is important for the optimal digestion [38]. Genetic variations in CFTR that affect membrane levels or channel activity led to various pancreatic phenotypes including chronic pancreatitis. Aberrant expression of CFTR causes to diminished fluid and HCO3– secretion leading to decreased intraluminal pH, decreased washout of the digestive enzymes, and more viscous protein rich ductal fluid. These changes promote the formation of intraluminal protein plugs [39, 40].

4.4 Oxidative distress

Moreover, a hypothesis is proposed which implies that mutation-induced misfolding, secretory blockage, and consequent endoplasmic reticulum (ER) stress can lead to acinar cell damage and pancreatitis [41]. Some of associated genes are CPA1 and CEL. Recent studies have also reported CLDN2, and MORC Family CW-Type Zinc Finger 4 (MORC4) gene are associated with CP, but the mechanism has not elicited, yet [4, 14].

Pathogenic CPA1 variants are detected both late but especially early onset CP due to proenzyme mis-folding, resulting in a secretion defect and intracellular retention [42, 43]. A deletion mutation in CEL is founded to cause an increasement in ER stress, through activation of the unfolded protein response and causing cell death by apoptosis [44].

The pancreas consists of three critical cell lineages: acinar, ductal and endocrine46. Adjacent to the acinar cells around small pancreatic ducts and blood vessels are pancreatic stellate cells, that compromise around 4–7% of all parenchymal cells [45, 46]. The hypotheses mentioned above lead to cellular injury, which turns into chronic inflammation and then eventually fibrosis.

As explained before, the secretory parenchyma but mainly the acinar cells are destroyed by processes such as toxification, inflammation, duct obstruction or oxidative stress. Increasing evidence indicates that pancreatic stellate cells (PSC) are the major mediators of fibrosis, resulting in the formation of extracellular matrix (ECM) in the organ. Fibrosis causes acinar cells and duct cells to injure and disappeared. This process ultimately leads to progressive loss of the lobular morphology and structure of the pancreas resulting in functional impairment of both exocrine and endocrine functions, eventually leading to clinical symptoms such as pain, malnutrition, or diabetes [47, 48]. Furthermore, the pancreatic stellate cells activate into myofibroblast-like phenotypes, proliferate, and secrete collagen I and III and fibronectin [49, 50]. Hence, the initial of the pancreas, leads to cell necrosis and/or apoptosis and consequently release of cytokines/growth factors (e.g., tumor growth factor b1, interleukin-8, platelet-derived growth factor and CC-chemokines), either from immigrating inflammatory cells, especially macrophages, and/or nearby preexistent epithelial or mesenchymal cells [51–54]. Thereafter damaged cells are phagocytosed by macrophages, causing release of cytokines, which in turn causes activation and proliferation of PCS [55]. So, a vicious circle of the irreversible event has started. These metalloproteinases are in return regulated by cytokine tumor growth factor (TGF)-β1s, which through autocrine inhibition enhances pancreatic fibrogenesis by reducing collagen degradation [50].

5. Diagnosis

The diagnosis of the chronic pancreatitis is still challenging especially in the early stages of the disease. Clinician must be suspected chronic pancreatitis in a patient with chronic abdominal pain (especially in upper quadrants), weight loss, steatorrhea, and endocrine pancreatic insufficiency. All patients with suspected chronic pancreatitis should have a dedicated pancreatic protocol to rule out pancreas carcinoma. Clinician should remember that any patient with chronic abdominal pain may also be had suffered from chronic abdominal pain syndrome, history of ERCP-related pancreatitis or any ductal changes. In most cases follow-up with serial imaging and physiological tests are recommended [56]. Once the diagnosis is confirmed, physician should characterize the etiology of chronic pancreatitis. TIGAR-O classification and modified MANNHEIM classification should be evaluated. TIGAR-O classification is a mnemonic for toxic metabolic, idiopathic, genetic mutations, autoimmune, recurrent, and severe acute pancreatitis associated chronic pancreatitis and obstructive etiologies [46]. Modified MANNHEIM classification is a mnemonic for multiple risk factors, alcohol consumption, nicotine consumption, nutritional factors (hyperlipidemia, hypertriglyceridemia), hereditary factors, efferent duct factors, immunologic factors, miscellaneous factors (hypercalcemia, hyperparathyroidism, chronic renal failure, toxins) [45].

Contrast-enhanced CT should be the initial diagnostic tool. CT scans have an overall sensitivity of 75% for chronic pancreatitis. Enlargement of the main duct (2–4 mm), glandular enlargement, heterogenous parenchyma, small (<10 mm) or lager (>10 mm) cavities, irregular ductal borders, irregular head/body contour and increased echogenicity of main duct wall are the probable pathologies that are seen in CT scan. After seeing these pathologies physician should suspect chronic pancreatitis and follow-up the patient. The other imaging technique for chronic pancreatitis is MRI and MRCP. Current MRI and MRCP technologies can provide high-quality images both parenchyma and ductal system [56]. T1 sequence in MRI is helpful for evaluating parenchymal changes in chronic pancreatitis. MRCP is used for evaluating ductal changes in chronic pancreatitis. Intravenous secretin administration during MRCP imaging stimulates pancreatic fluid secretion and can improve the visualization of ductal tree [57]. The other imaging technique for evaluating chronic pancreatitis is ultrasonography and endoscopic ultrasonography (EUS). EUS finding can be classified as two subgroups which are parenchymal features and ductal features [58]. EUS is one of the most promising imaging techniques for diagnosis and evaluating chronic pancreatitis. However, the EUS imaging needs experienced clinician. EUS is now considered to be the most sensitive CP diagnostic investigation, especially in the early stages of the disease [59, 60].

Blood amylase and lipase levels can help the physician to diagnose acute pancreatitis however, in chronic pancreatitis these levels often normal. The diagnosis of the chronic pancreatitis with blood tests are challenging. There can be some clues like hypertriglyceridemia, hypercalcemia, hyperparathyroidism and hyperlipidemia. On the other hand, fecal elastase levels are often decreased in chronic pancreatitis. Also, diagnosis of type 3c diabetes (defined as pancreatic islet dysfunction and islet loss due to diseases of endocrine pancreas) is helpful for diagnosing the disease. Increased levels of hemoglobin A1c (HbA1c), absence of insulin resistance, loss of incretin secretion and low levels of fat-soluble vitamin concentrations can support the diagnosis of the chronic pancreatitis. The secretin stimulation test can be used with MRCP and for research. Secretin stimulation test is a complex procedure. Firstly, the physician takes a sample from duodenal fluid as a baseline enzyme value then performs intravenous secretin administration after that the second sampling from duodenal fluid is done. Fecal elastase levels and secretin stimulation test results show the damage of exocrine pancreas.

6. Clinical presentation

The most common symptom of chronic pancreatitis is abdominal pain which is present more than 80% of patients. The pain is commonly described as a dull pain in the epigastrium radiating to the back that worsens after meals. The character, pattern and intensity of pain can vary among patients and does not correlate with the extent of pathological/morphologic changes [61]. Patients with alcohol related CP are more likely to experience pain, whereas late-onset CP is stated to be less painful [62]. Nausea, vomiting or both may accompany pain during exacerbations of pain attacks or during episodes of acute pancreatitis. Approximately 70% of adult patients with CP experience at least 1 episode of acute pancreatitis and 50% have recurrent pancreatitis during the clinical course of the disease [63].

Several anatomical complications can occur in CP due to local inflammation or glandular fibrosis symptoms. The formation of pancreatic pseudocysts, which can occur in 10–40% of patients during their lifetime, is one of the most frequent anatomic complications. Pseudocysts can cause gastroduodenal outlet obstruction and/or biliary obstruction, depending on their anatomic location and size [64].

Other anatomical complications are pancreatic stones, pancreatic strictures, biliary strictures and thrombosis of splanchnic vasculature.

One of the complications of CP is exocrine pancreatic insufficiency (EPI). EPI is a condition characterized by insufficient production and/or secretion of pancreatic enzymes for the digestion of nutrients. The predominant symptoms of EPI are related to fat malabsorption. Mild EPI can cause abdominal bloating and discomfort, while severe EPI can cause overt steatorrhea, weight loss and fat-soluble vitamin deficiencies. Generally, EPI does not develop for more than a decade after disease onset, due to the exceptional reserve of the exocrine pancreas and the redundant pathways for digestion of proteins and carbohydrates. Although prevalence of EPI at diagnosis of CP is 10–13%. EPI affects more than 70% of patients with CP throughout their lifespan and is especially frequent in those with proximal obstruction of the pancreatic duct or a history of pancreatic resection [64, 65].

Another complication of CP is metabolic bone disorder which has also been referred to as CP-associated osteopathy. A meta-analysis estimated that the pooled prevalence of osteoporosis was 23.4% and of osteopenia, 39.8% [66]. Additionally, patients with CP have a higher risk of low trauma fractures (vertebrae, hip, and wrist) and the risk of fractures in patients with CP was similar to other gastrointestinal diseases, such as cirrhosis, celiac disease and history of gastrectomy [67].

Diabetes mellitus (DM) is a frequent complication of CP. Prevalence of endocrine insufficiency at diagnosis of CP is 10–33% [4, 8]. A recent systematic review identified a 15% prevalence of new onset diabetes within 36 months and a 33% prevalence within 60 months of CP diagnosis [68]. DM usually occurs several years after the onset of the disease and can eventually affect up to 80% of patients over their lifespan [69]. Due to the high prevalence of CP-DM, annual screening for DM is recommended [70, 71]. In a recent study of participants with CP, DM was more likely to occur in participants who were older, obese, male, black race, or had a family history of DM and factors independently associated with DM included both obesity and the presence of exocrine pancreatic insufficiency [72]. A prolonged period of CP, the absence of pain, cigarette smoking, and an increase in visceral adipose tissue have all been linked to CP-DM [73, 74].

7. Medical treatment of the pain

Chronic Pancreatitis related pain is typically among the most severe pain of all chronic diseases and has a major impact on quality of life and disability [16, 17]. That is why pain control plays a key role in the treatment of CP. Combinations of medical, endoscopic, and surgical approaches may be used to relieve abdominal pain in patients with CP [75, 76].

All patients having pain should be offered medical management. Patients with inflammatory mass, pancreatic duct obstruction due to stricture and/or main duct stones or peripancreatic complications (e.g. pseudocyst) may require additional interventions. Even in patients who tend to be suitable for endoscopic or surgical therapy, initial medical management of pain is advised to provide relief, greater understanding of the mechanism of pain, response to treatment, and if there is any significant sensitization [77].

The World Health Organization analgesic ladder for cancer pain is widely used by physicians to treat CP pain as there are no recommendations for the choice, usage and dosage of analgesics [78]. This stepwise approach recommends acetaminophen and nonsteroidal anti-inflammatory drugs (e.g., diclofenac, ibuprofen, and naproxen) as initial choice. When patient has constant and/or severe pain that cannot be controlled with non-narcotic analgesics, narcotic medications can be used. The first option of narcotics should be a weaker, mixed agonist–antagonist or partial agonist (e.g., tramadol) prior to the use of stronger narcotics (e.g., morphine, hydrocodone and hydromorphone). If opioids are needed, they should be administered orally in a long-acting form -lancet). Physicians must be aware of their side effects (e.g., constipation, nausea, sedation, increased risk of falls, and risk of dependence and substance misuse) and capable of managing them. That is why, patients that are likely to undergo long-term narcotic analgesia for pancreatic pain are most effectively assessed and treated at a pain clinic [77].

Because of these adverse effects of opioids, co-analgesics should also be tried, and interventional therapy (such as surgery) should be considered before starting opioids. Co-analgesics such as antidepressants and anticonvulsants (gabapentin, pregabalin) have been shown to be beneficial in the treatment of chronic visceral and neuropathic pain in chronic pancreatitis and can help to minimize the need for opioids [62, 79]. Pregabalin is shown to have better efficacy in decreasing daily pain scores than placebo, however central nervous symptoms were seen in significant number of participants on pregabalin, potentially limiting its clinical usefulness [80]. Alternative analgesics such as esketamine are currently being investigated for this indication [61].

Antioxidant supplementation in may be beneficial especially for those patients with nonalcoholic-derived CP but additional trials are needed [81–83]. A randomized control study showed that pain relief significantly higher in the antioxidant group than in the placebo group [84].

8. Endoscopic treatment of the CP

Unfortunately, 30 and 60% of all patients ultimately require intervention. Endoscopic interventions have an important place for both in the diagnosing/staging of the disease and in the management of the CP complications [85].

8.1 Treatment of the pain

Although all therapeutic approaches for pancreatic pain is not very effective, endoscopic therapy is still one of the choices in patients whose pain is refractory to non-interventional therapy and who has remarkable anatomic alterations in their pancreas and/or in the surrounding tissue. There is no evidence for the use of the endoscopy in the mild disease or in painless CP [86–88]. Endoscopic therapy could be beneficial in patients with a symptomatic pancreatic duct obstruction in the pancreatic head or neck, together with an upstream duct dilatation, Plastic stents and fully covered self-expandable metal or biodegradable stents are safe and effective options for the relief of pancreatic outflow obstruction, and eventually of the pain [89–91]. Although celiac plexus (endoscopic or percutaneous) is still commonly used in clinical practice, the evidence for its efficacy of celiac plexus block in CP remains weak [92].

8.2 Treatment of the pancreatic duct stones

Pancreatic stones are the result of the CP and they are usually getting calcified with progression of the disease [93]. Pancreatic ductal stones which cause symptoms such as pain by obstructing the flow of pancreatic juice, recurrent episodes of pancreatitis, or present with pseudocyst or fistula and other complications can be treated by endoscopic methods [94].

The location of the stone in the duct and its number is important for deciding endoscopic methods. Stones in the head and neck of the pancreas can be extracted with endoscopy, with or without stent replacement. However, endoscopic treatment is not suitable for stones, which already caused overt local complications or are located distally [85, 95, 96].

Pancreatic duct stones smaller than 5 mm are extracted by the ERCP, while extracorporeal shock wave lithotripsy (ESWL) is suggested for the clearance of radiopaque obstructive stones larger than 5 mm. Furthermore, recent studies suggest that performance of ESWL prior to the endoscopic attempt at stone extraction can provide more successful stone clearance [97–99].

8.3 Treatment of the pancreatic pseudocyst

Pancreatic pseudocysts develop as a frequent complication between 20 and 40% of CP patients [100]. It is most prevalent in alcoholic CP, followed by idiopathic CP [101, 102]. Almost 40% of the pseudocyst, especially smaller ones can resolve within the 6 weeks after the attack. However, if it does not, the probability for a complication such as infection or rupture is 2/3 of all cases. Endoscopic drainage, which has a lower morbidity rate than surgery, is a successful treatment strategy for a symptomatic or complicated pseudocyst [103]. There are two main technics for the drainage of the pseudocyst: transmural or transpapillary drainage. Whereas transmural drainage can be applied to every pseudocyst, transpapillary drainage is feasible, only if the pseudocyst has a connection to major pancreatic duct [104]. It is recommended that EUS- guided access has higher technical success than the conventional approach [105]. Another important consideration when planning a pseudocyst drainage is the existence of pseudoaneurysms and portal hypertension. EUS guided drainage is recommended in case of portal hypertension as bleeding is common complication in these patients [106]. And since the mortality is very high due to ruptured aneurysms, embolization of the artery prior to the endoscopic intervention is recommended [107].

8.4 Treatment of the biliary strictures

Biliary strictures are big obstacles during CP treatment. They are prevalent almost 46% of the CP patients. The symptoms include abdominal pain, jaundice, fever and the laboratory results show elevated serum alkaline phosphatase and/or bilirubin [108]. The endoscopic therapy is found to be long term effective only in 1/3 of the endoscopically treated patients. Therefore, endoscopic management is mostly used as transient therapy before the surgery [109, 110]. Studies suggest that placement of multiple plastic stents into the bile duct to treat bile duct obstruction in patients with chronic pancreatitis [111]. An important point about this clinical picture is absolute exclusion of the malignancy. It is essential to exchange the stents every 3 months to prevent the occlusion. However, this period is not such critical in multiple stents [111].

9. Surgical treatment

When medical treatments fail, endoscopy and surgical resection, drainage procedures, or both can be used to relieve pain. These procedures are used to treat pancreatic ductal obstruction caused by stones, strictures, or both in order to relieve intraductal hypertension and thereby pain [112]. Whether surgical or endoscopic therapy should be offered first is controversial [2].

Despite weaknesses in the study design, two randomized controlled trials found that surgery offered greater long-term pain relief than endoscopy [95, 96, 113]. This effect may be explained by the fact that surgical treatment not only relieves ductal hypertension by allowing drainage, but also removes inflamed tissue that causes neural changes and pain [114, 115]. In another clinical trial, comparing the cost-effectiveness of endoscopy and surgery, 38 CP patients were equally randomized and the mean number of ERCPs performed in the endoscopy group (6.3 vs. 0.4) was higher than in the surgery group [116].

Many patients prefer endoscopic therapy at first, in spite of the efficacy of surgery and frequent need for repeated procedures among people undergoing endoscopy because it is less invasive [112]. Patients with large inflammatory mass of the pancreatic head, distal pancreatic stenosis, and pancreatic head calcifications can be challenging to treat by endoscopy [85]. If endotherapy fails to provide immediate symptom relief without the need for repeated endoscopies, surgery should be considered by a multidisciplinary team [2]. Endoscopy is most frequently used as a therapeutic trial to determine patients most likely to benefit from surgery. While this approach is intuitive, the clinical evidence supporting this approach is not robust and more methods for predicting pain response are urgently required to prevent unhelpful interventions [117].

Surgery can be an effective first-line treatment for patients with CP who have large and multiple pancreatic stones or complicated strictures, an inflammatory mass of the head or a disease confined to the pancreatic tail [112]. Patients who are referred within 3–5 years of the onset of symptoms and have had less than four endoscopic procedures prior to surgery have better surgical outcomes [118].

The type of surgery is determined by the anatomy, the course of the disease, and local preferences [119]. The surgical approaches used to treat patients with CP are drainage options, resection options and neuroablative procedures [120]. Drainage options are cystojejunostomy, laterolateral pancreaticojejunostomy (Partington-Rochelle procedure) and caudal drainage (Puestow procedure). Resection options are pancreaticoduodenectomy (PD/Kausch-Whipple procedure) or pylorus preserving pancreaticoduodenectomy (PPPD/Traverso-Longmire-procedure), duodenum-preserving pancreatic head resection (DPPHR (Beger, Frey, Hamburg, Berne)), V-shaped excision, segmental resection and distal/total pancreatectomy. Neuroablative procedures are percutaneous radiofrequency ablation of the splanchnic nerves and thoracoscopic splanchnicectomy [120].

Total pancreatectomy accompanied by digestion of the pancreas, isolation of the islet cells and infusion into the patient's portal circulation is a radical surgical alternative that enables glucose homeostasis to be maintained without the need for immunosuppression of allogeneic islet transplantation [121]. Outside of the United States, total pancreatectomy with autoislet transplantation is still not widely available [2]. The primary indication for total pancreatectomy and islet auto transplantation is intractable pain that has a significant effect on quality of life (TPIAT) according to current clinical guidelines [122]. The procedure is successful in reducing or eliminating pain with a positive impact on quality of life [121–123]. However, severe pain persists in a large number of patients even after total pancreatectomy [124].

10. Treatment of endocrine insufficiency/CP-related DM

CP-related DM (CP-DM) is the most frequent cause of pancreatogenic DM (which has also been referred to as type 3c DM). Biannual fasting glucose and glycated hemoglobin should be obtained to assess for diabetes in CP patients [70]. The management of type 3c diabetes follows general recommendations for diabetics.

A healthy lifestyle with regular exercise and a balanced diet should accompany medical treatment. Optimized pancreatic enzyme replacement therapy improves duodenal sensing and uptake of complex nutrients, thus stabilizes blood sugar levels. Due to a lack of counter regulation, patients with type 3c diabetes have an increased risk for hypoglycemia and should be counseled accordingly. The treatment of choice is often insulin, but in mild hyperglycemia (HbA1c <8%) metformin has also been recommended [2]. In addition to its glucose lowering effect, a meta-analysis of 12 observational studies showed that metformin reduced the risk of pancreatic cancer development in people with diabetes [125]. Sulfonylureas should be avoided. Although glinides, thiazolidinediones, α-glycosidase inhibitors, incretin-based therapies, and SGLT2 inhibitors have not been tested in randomized trials, they may be effective in certain cases [61]. In order to understand the pathogenesis better and to inform the prevention and treatment of CP-DM, a detailed characterization of changes in glucose homeostasis in CP DM compared to type 2 DM is required [61].

11. Treatment of exocrine pancreatic insufficiency

The assessment of functional deficiencies should be part of the initial evaluation and monitoring of patients with CP. Exocrine pancreatic insufficiency (EPI) is indicated by symptoms of steatorrhea (foul-smelling, oily stool), diarrhea, and weight loss. The gold standard for the diagnosis of EPI is a decreased coefficient of fat absorption (CFA) [1]. CFA of less than 93% (or >7 g of fat per 24 hours from a 72-hour fecal fat collection in a patient who is consuming 100 g of dietary fat each day during stool collection) defines steatorrhea or fat malabsorption [112]. Although this is a highly accurate test for fat malabsorption, it is rarely used in clinical practice because it is difficult for patients to perform properly. Several other indirect measures (e.g. fecal elastase (FE-1), serum trypsin) and clear tests (endoscopic secretin) are used to diagnose exocrine insufficiency [126]. The accuracy of these tests is highest in the presence of severe exocrine insufficiency (defined as steatorrhea). FE −1 is an indirect measure of exocrine function that is performed on a random stool sample. Since false positive test results are common due to diarrhea, the fecal elastase-1 test should not be used to evaluate patients with unexplained diarrhea [127]. Furthermore, the sensitivity and specificity of this test is open to discuss [126]. Shortly, there are no established criterion standard for mild to moderate exocrine insufficiency. The lack of a reliable and easy test to diagnose and monitor the treatment of EPI remains one of the biggest challenges for the management of EPI. All patients with chronic pancreatitis and pancreatic exocrine insufficiency, or signs of malnutrition should be treated with 40,000–50,000 lipase units of pancreatic enzymes per meal, and dose should be increased until symptoms are relieved [2]. In patients with EPI with persistent symptoms despite pancreatic enzyme replacement therapy (PERT) initiation, additional treatment strategies to consider are increase in the dosage of PERT, addition of a proton pump inhibitor (if not currently used), consideration of alternative etiologies of symptoms in CP, such as small intestinal bacterial overgrowth or lactose intolerance, and consideration of other causes of fat malabsorption [128]. According to a large randomized controlled trial in unselected noncritically ill inpatients, nutritional evaluation and treatment can reduce morbidity and mortality [129].

12. Treatment of metabolic bone disorder

The high prevalence of CP-related osteopathy can be partly explained by common risk factors such as cigarette smoking and heavy alcohol consumption.

Furthermore, chronic inflammation caused by CP is likely to contribute to a pro-inflammatory environment that leads to net bone loss [130]. Ultimately, patients with CP are at high risk of vitamin D deficiency, especially when EPI is present [131].

CP-associated osteopathy management follows general treatment guidelines, including calcium and vitamin D supplementation, weight-bearing exercises, and smoking cessation. Oral bisphosphonate therapy, when indicated, should be closely monitored to ensure that patients tolerate it. If patient cannot tolerate it, switching to an alternative anti-resorptive therapies should be considered. Lastly, uncontrolled data indicates that PERT could potentially reduce the risk of fractures in subjects with CP, but further studies are required before this can be universally recommended [132].

In other gastrointestinal conditions, such as celiac disease, cholestatic liver disease, and inflammatory bowel disease, baseline screening with a DEXA scan has been widely adopted. That is why, baseline screening with DEXA in CP is reasonable considering that CP has higher odds of fractures compared with other gastrointestinal conditions [67, 71].

13. CP and pancreatic cancer surveillance

Pancreatic cancer is expected to be the second to third most common cause of cancer-related deaths by 2030 due to late diagnosis and inadequate treatment choices [133]. The relationship between chronic pancreatitis and pancreatic cancer is complicated since common risk factors and the course of the disease affect the rate of malignant transformation [2]. Epidemiological studies have consistently demonstrated an increased risk of pancreatic cancer (i.e., pancreatic ductal adenocarcinoma) in patients with CP, which is thought to be a result of chronic inflammation leading to hyperproliferation of pancreatic stellate cells [134]. In a meta-analysis, the risk of developing pancreatic cancer is increased in patients with chronic pancreatitis, but this is potentially confounded by smoking, which is an independent risk factor [135, 136].

Patients with hereditary pancreatitis have a 70-fold increased risk of developing pancreatic cancer compared to the control population [137, 138]. Patients with tropical pancreatitis can have a relative risk of more than 100; however, recent updates are required to see if there has been a similar decline over time [139].

Patients with hereditary chronic pancreatitis should be screened starting at age 40 or 20 years after the diagnosis of chronic pancreatitis, regardless of gene carrier status.

While PDAC screening is not routinely recommended, it is advised to retain high clinical suspicion in those with unexplained symptoms, such as unexplained weight loss or changes in abdominal pain characteristics [1, 71]. In all patients with chronic pancreatitis, newly diagnosed diabetes may be an early sign of pancreatic cancer and may prompt further research. Unfortunately, the baseline morphological changes in the pancreas (especially the main pancreatic duct dilatation) in CP make it difficult to recognize a small neoplasm in cross-sectional imaging. In patients with multiple calcifications which may mask changes in the parenchyma, there is a chance of sampling error with EUS-guided fine needle aspiration [1].

14. Conclusion

CP is a multifactorial disease resulting in fibroinflammatory changes, endocrine and exocrine dysfunction of the pancreas. Although some etiologic factors such as alcohol, hereditary changes are well established, idiopathic cases constitute a considerable percentage. Both the endoscopic and radiologic techniques are helping the clinicians for diagnosing the disease. Medical, endoscopic and surgical treatment options are also effective and long-lasting. The main challenge in the field is early diagnosis of the CP before the symptoms exaggerate and staging the disease to monitor and treat the patients in a more appropriate way. Therefore, future prospective clinical trials and translational studies in search of novel diagnostic markers and staging methods are absolutely needed.

Author details

Didem Saka[1], Can Boynukara[1], Elif Reyyan Çadırcıbaşı[1] and Gürhan Şişman[2]*

1 School of Medicine, Acıbadem Mehmet Ali Aydınlar University, İstanbul, Turkey

2 Department of Gastroenterology, Acıbadem Mehmet Ali Aydınlar University, İstanbul, Turkey

*Address all correspondence to: gurhan.sisman@acibadem.edu.tr

References

[1] Hart PA, Conwell DL. Chronic Pancreatitis: Managing a Difficult Disease. Am J Gastroenterol. 2020;115(1):49-55.

[2] Beyer G, Habtezion A, Werner J, Lerch MM, Mayerle J. Chronic pancreatitis. Lancet. 2020;396(10249): 499-512.

[3] Conwell DL, Banks PA, Sandhu BS, Sherman S, Al-Kaade S, Gardner TB, et al. Validation of Demographics, Etiology, and Risk Factors for Chronic Pancreatitis in the USA: A Report of the North American Pancreas Study (NAPS) Group. Dig Dis Sci. 2017;62(8):2133-40.

[4] Whitcomb DC, LaRusch J, Krasinskas AM, Klei L, Smith JP, Brand RE, et al. Common genetic variants in the CLDN2 and PRSS1-PRSS2 loci alter risk for alcohol-related and sporadic pancreatitis. Nat Genet. 2012;44(12):1349-54.

[5] Peery AF, Crockett SD, Murphy CC, Lund JL, Dellon ES, Williams JL, et al. Burden and Cost of Gastrointestinal, Liver, and Pancreatic Diseases in the United States: Update 2018. Gastroenterology. 2019;156(1): 254-72.e11.

[6] Sankaran SJ, Xiao AY, Wu LM, Windsor JA, Forsmark CE, Petrov MS. Frequency of progression from acute to chronic pancreatitis and risk factors: a meta-analysis. Gastroenterology. 2015;149(6):1490-500.e1.

[7] Ahmed Ali U, Issa Y, Hagenaars JC, Bakker OJ, van Goor H, Nieuwenhuijs VB, et al. Risk of Recurrent Pancreatitis and Progression to Chronic Pancreatitis After a First Episode of Acute Pancreatitis. Clin Gastroenterol Hepatol. 2016;14(5): 738-46.

[8] Hori Y, Vege SS, Chari ST, Gleeson FC, Levy MJ, Pearson RK, et al. Classic chronic pancreatitis is associated with prior acute pancreatitis in only 50% of patients in a large single-institution study. Pancreatology. 2019;19(2):224-9.

[9] Wilcox CM, Sandhu BS, Singh V, Gelrud A, Abberbock JN, Sherman S, et al. Racial Differences in the Clinical Profile, Causes, and Outcome of Chronic Pancreatitis. Am J Gastroenterol. 2016;111(10):1488-96.

[10] Şişman G, Köroğlu E, Erzin Y, Hatemi İ, Tuncer M, Şentürk H. Demographic characteristics of chronic pancreatitis patients in the era of endosonography: Experience of a single tertiary referral center in Turkey. Turk J Gastroenterol. 2016;27(3):284-9.

[11] Irving HM, Samokhvalov AV, Rehm J. Alcohol as a risk factor for pancreatitis. A systematic review and meta-analysis. Jop. 2009;10(4):387-92.

[12] Yadav D, Hawes RH, Brand RE, Anderson MA, Money ME, Banks PA, et al. Alcohol consumption, cigarette smoking, and the risk of recurrent acute and chronic pancreatitis. Arch Intern Med. 2009;169(11):1035-45.

[13] Xue J, Zhao Q, Sharma V, Nguyen LP, Lee YN, Pham KL, et al. Aryl Hydrocarbon Receptor Ligands in Cigarette Smoke Induce Production of Interleukin-22 to Promote Pancreatic Fibrosis in Models of Chronic Pancreatitis. Gastroenterology. 2016;151(6):1206-17.

[14] Giri AK, Midha S, Banerjee P, Agrawal A, Mehdi SJ, Dhingra R, et al. Common Variants in CLDN2 and MORC4 Genes Confer Disease Susceptibility in Patients with Chronic Pancreatitis. PLoS One. 2016;11(1): e0147345.

[15] V K. Robins basic pathology e-book. AK A, editor. Elsevier Health Sciences2017.

[16] Gardner TB, Kennedy AT, Gelrud A, Banks PA, Vege SS, Gordon SR, et al. Chronic pancreatitis and its effect on employment and health care experience: results of a prospective American multicenter study. Pancreas. 2010;39(4):498-501.

[17] Gukovskaya AS, Mouria M, Gukovsky I, Reyes CN, Kasho VN, Faller LD, et al. Ethanol metabolism and transcription factor activation in pancreatic acinar cells in rats. Gastroenterology. 2002;122(1): 106-18.

[18] Grauvogel J, Grauvogel TD, Gebhard MM, Werner J. Combined effects of chronic and acute ethanol on pancreatic injury and microcirculation. Pancreas. 2012;41(5):717-23.

[19] Vonlaufen A, Wilson JS, Pirola RC, Apte MV. Role of alcohol metabolism in chronic pancreatitis. Alcohol Res Health. 2007;30(1):48-54.

[20] Gu H, Werner J, Bergmann F, Whitcomb DC, Büchler MW, Fortunato F. Necro-inflammatory response of pancreatic acinar cells in the pathogenesis of acute alcoholic pancreatitis. Cell Death Dis. 2013;4(10):e816.

[21] Apte MV, Wilson JS. Stellate cell activation in alcoholic pancreatitis. Pancreas. 2003;27(4):316-20.

[22] Sendler M, van den Brandt C, Glaubitz J, Wilden A, Golchert J, Weiss FU, et al. NLRP3 Inflammasome Regulates Development of Systemic Inflammatory Response and Compensatory Anti-Inflammatory Response Syndromes in Mice With Acute Pancreatitis. Gastroenterology. 2020;158(1):253-69.e14.

[23] Xue J, Sharma V, Hsieh MH, Chawla A, Murali R, Pandol SJ, et al. Alternatively activated macrophages promote pancreatic fibrosis in chronic pancreatitis. Nat Commun. 2015;6:7158.

[24] Alahmari AA, Sreekumar B, Patel V, Ashat M, Alexandre M, Uduman AK, et al. Cigarette toxin 4-(methylnitrosamino)-1-(3-pyridyl)-1-butanone (NNK) induces experimental pancreatitis through α7 nicotinic acetylcholine receptors (nAChRs) in mice. PLoS One. 2018;13(6):e0197362.

[25] Rinderknecht H. Activation of pancreatic zymogens. Normal activation, premature intrapancreatic activation, protective mechanisms against inappropriate activation. Dig Dis Sci. 1986;31(3):314-21.

[26] Mayerle J, Sendler M, Hegyi E, Beyer G, Lerch MM, Sahin-Tóth M. Genetics, Cell Biology, and Pathophysiology of Pancreatitis. Gastroenterology. 2019;156(7): 1951-68.e1.

[27] Hegyi E, Sahin-Tóth M. Genetic Risk in Chronic Pancreatitis: The Trypsin-Dependent Pathway. Dig Dis Sci. 2017;62(7):1692-701.

[28] Nemoda Z, Sahin-Tóth M. Chymotrypsin C (caldecrin) stimulates autoactivation of human cationic trypsinogen. J Biol Chem. 2006;281(17):11879-86.

[29] Szabó A, Sahin-Tóth M. Increased activation of hereditary pancreatitis-associated human cationic trypsinogen mutants in presence of chymotrypsin C. J Biol Chem. 2012;287(24):20701-10.

[30] Witt H, Sahin-Tóth M, Landt O, Chen JM, Kähne T, Drenth JP, et al. A degradation-sensitive anionic trypsinogen (PRSS2) variant protects against chronic pancreatitis. Nat Genet. 2006;38(6):668-73.

[31] Aoun E, Chang CC, Greer JB, Papachristou GI, Barmada MM, Whitcomb DC. Pathways to injury in chronic pancreatitis: decoding the role of the high-risk SPINK1 N34S haplotype using meta-analysis. PLoS One. 2008;3(4):e2003.

[32] Zhou J, Sahin-Tóth M. Chymotrypsin C mutations in chronic pancreatitis. J Gastroenterol Hepatol. 2011;26(8):1238-46.

[33] Szmola R, Bence M, Carpentieri A, Szabó A, Costello CE, Samuelson J, et al. Chymotrypsin C is a co-activator of human pancreatic procarboxypeptidases A1 and A2. J Biol Chem. 2011;286(3):1819-27.

[34] Rosendahl J, Kirsten H, Hegyi E, Kovacs P, Weiss FU, Laumen H, et al. Genome-wide association study identifies inversion in the CTRB1-CTRB2 locus to modify risk for alcoholic and non-alcoholic chronic pancreatitis. Gut. 2018;67(10):1855-63.

[35] Moore PC, Cortez JT, Chamberlain CE, Alba D, Berger AC, Quandt Z, et al. Elastase 3B mutation links to familial pancreatitis with diabetes and pancreatic adenocarcinoma. J Clin Invest. 2019;129(11):4676-81.

[36] Klöppel G, Detlefsen S, Feyerabend B. Fibrosis of the pancreas: the initial tissue damage and the resulting pattern. Virchows Arch. 2004;445(1):1-8.

[37] AA A. Pathogenesis of Chronic Pancreatitis. Pancreapedia: Exocrine Pancreas Knowledge Base2016.

[38] Hegyi P, Wilschanski M, Muallem S, Lukacs GL, Sahin-Tóth M, Uc A, et al. CFTR: A New Horizon in the Pathomechanism and Treatment of Pancreatitis. Rev Physiol Biochem Pharmacol. 2016;170:37-66.

[39] Ko SB, Azuma S, Yoshikawa T, Yamamoto A, Kyokane K, Ko MS, et al. Molecular mechanisms of pancreatic stone formation in chronic pancreatitis. Front Physiol. 2012;3:415.

[40] Sarles H, Sarles JC, Camatte R, Muratore R, Gaini M, Guien C, et al. Observations on 205 confirmed cases of acute pancreatitis, recurring pancreatitis, and chronic pancreatitis. Gut. 1965;6(6):545-59.

[41] Sahin-Tóth M. Genetic risk in chronic pancreatitis: the misfolding-dependent pathway. Curr Opin Gastroenterol. 2017;33(5):390-5.

[42] Witt H, Beer S, Rosendahl J, Chen JM, Chandak GR, Masamune A, et al. Variants in CPA1 are strongly associated with early onset chronic pancreatitis. Nat Genet. 2013;45(10): 1216-20.

[43] Kujko AA, Berki DM, Oracz G, Wejnarska K, Antoniuk J, Wertheim-Tysarowska K, et al. A novel p.Ser282Pro CPA1 variant is associated with autosomal dominant hereditary pancreatitis. Gut. 662017. p. 1728-30.

[44] Xiao X, Jones G, Sevilla WA, Stolz DB, Magee KE, Haughney M, et al. A Carboxyl Ester Lipase (CEL) Mutant Causes Chronic Pancreatitis by Forming Intracellular Aggregates That Activate Apoptosis. J Biol Chem. 2016;291(44):23224-36.

[45] Schneider A, Löhr JM, Singer MV. The M-ANNHEIM classification of chronic pancreatitis: introduction of a unifying classification system based on a review of previous classifications of the disease. J Gastroenterol. 2007;42(2):101-19.

[46] Etemad B, Whitcomb DC. Chronic pancreatitis: diagnosis, classification, and new genetic developments. Gastroenterology. 2001;120(3): 682-707.

[47] Lévy P, Barthet M, Mollard BR, Amouretti M, Marion-Audibert AM, Dyard F. Estimation of the prevalence and incidence of chronic pancreatitis and its complications. Gastroenterol Clin Biol. 2006;30(6-7):838-44.

[48] Andrén-Sandberg A, Hoem D, Gislason H. Pain management in chronic pancreatitis. Eur J Gastroenterol Hepatol. 2002;14(9):957-70.

[49] Apte MV, Haber PS, Darby SJ, Rodgers SC, McCaughan GW, Korsten MA, et al. Pancreatic stellate cells are activated by proinflammatory cytokines: implications for pancreatic fibrogenesis. Gut. 1999;44(4):534-41.

[50] Shek FW, Benyon RC, Walker FM, McCrudden PR, Pender SL, Williams EJ, et al. Expression of transforming growth factor-beta 1 by pancreatic stellate cells and its implications for matrix secretion and turnover in chronic pancreatitis. Am J Pathol. 2002;160(5):1787-98.

[51] Andoh A, Takaya H, Saotome T, Shimada M, Hata K, Araki Y, et al. Cytokine regulation of chemokine (IL-8, MCP-1, and RANTES) gene expression in human pancreatic periacinar myofibroblasts. Gastroenterology. 2000;119(1):211-9.

[52] Ebert M, Kasper HU, Hernberg S, Friess H, Büchler MW, Roessner A, et al. Overexpression of platelet-derived growth factor (PDGF) B chain and type beta PDGF receptor in human chronic pancreatitis. Dig Dis Sci. 1998;43(3):567-74.

[53] Luttenberger T, Schmid-Kotsas A, Menke A, Siech M, Beger H, Adler G, et al. Platelet-derived growth factors stimulate proliferation and extracellular matrix synthesis of pancreatic stellate cells: implications in pathogenesis of pancreas fibrosis. Lab Invest. 2000;80(1):47-55.

[54] Saurer L, Reber P, Schaffner T, Büchler MW, Buri C, Kappeler A, et al. Differential expression of chemokines in normal pancreas and in chronic pancreatitis. Gastroenterology. 2000;118(2):356-67.

[55] Haber PS, Keogh GW, Apte MV, Moran CS, Stewart NL, Crawford DH, et al. Activation of pancreatic stellate cells in human and experimental pancreatic fibrosis. Am J Pathol. 1999;155(4):1087-95.

[56] Conwell DL, Lee LS, Yadav D, Longnecker DS, Miller FH, Mortele KJ, et al. American Pancreatic Association Practice Guidelines in Chronic Pancreatitis: evidence-based report on diagnostic guidelines. Pancreas. 2014;43(8):1143-62.

[57] Zhang L, Chari S, Smyrk TC, Deshpande V, Klöppel G, Kojima M, et al. Autoimmune pancreatitis (AIP) type 1 and type 2: an international consensus study on histopathologic diagnostic criteria. Pancreas. 2011;40(8):1172-9.

[58] Gardner TB, Taylor DJ, Gordon SR. Reported findings on endoscopic ultrasound examinations for chronic pancreatitis: toward establishing an endoscopic ultrasound quality benchmark. Pancreas. 2014;43(1):37-40.

[59] Löhr JM, Dominguez-Munoz E, Rosendahl J, Besselink M, Mayerle J, Lerch MM, et al. United European Gastroenterology evidence-based guidelines for the diagnosis and therapy of chronic pancreatitis (HaPanEU). United European Gastroenterol J. 2017;5(2):153-99.

[60] Iglesias-García J, Lindkvist B, Lariño-Noia J, Domínguez-Muñoz JE. The role of EUS in relation to other imaging modalities in the differential diagnosis between mass forming chronic pancreatitis, autoimmune pancreatitis and ductal pancreatic

adenocarcinoma. Rev Esp Enferm Dig. 2012;104(6):315-21.

[61] Wilcox CM, Yadav D, Ye T, Gardner TB, Gelrud A, Sandhu BS, et al. Chronic pancreatitis pain pattern and severity are independent of abdominal imaging findings. Clin Gastroenterol Hepatol. 2015;13(3):552-60; quiz e28-9.

[62] Drewes AM, Bouwense SAW, Campbell CM, Ceyhan GO, Delhaye M, Demir IE, et al. Guidelines for the understanding and management of pain in chronic pancreatitis. Pancreatology. 2017;17(5):720-31.

[63] Schwarzenberg SJ, Uc A, Zimmerman B, Wilschanski M, Wilcox CM, Whitcomb DC, et al. Chronic Pancreatitis: Pediatric and Adult Cohorts Show Similarities in Disease Progress Despite Different Risk Factors. J Pediatr Gastroenterol Nutr. 2019;68(4):566-73.

[64] Machicado JD, Chari ST, Timmons L, Tang G, Yadav D. A population-based evaluation of the natural history of chronic pancreatitis. Pancreatology. 2018;18(1):39-45.

[65] Layer P, Yamamoto H, Kalthoff L, Clain JE, Bakken LJ, DiMagno EP. The different courses of early- and late-onset idiopathic and alcoholic chronic pancreatitis. Gastroenterology. 1994;107(5):1481-7.

[66] Duggan SN, Smyth ND, Murphy A, Macnaughton D, O'Keefe SJ, Conlon KC. High prevalence of osteoporosis in patients with chronic pancreatitis: a systematic review and meta-analysis. Clin Gastroenterol Hepatol. 2014;12(2):219-28.

[67] Tignor AS, Wu BU, Whitlock TL, Lopez R, Repas K, Banks PA, et al. High prevalence of low-trauma fracture in chronic pancreatitis. Am J Gastroenterol. 2010;105(12):2680-6.

[68] Zhu X, Liu D, Wei Q, Lin H, Zhi M, Chen Y, et al. New-Onset Diabetes Mellitus After Chronic Pancreatitis Diagnosis: A Systematic Review and Meta-analysis. Pancreas. 2019;48(7):868-75.

[69] Hart PA, Bellin MD, Andersen DK, Bradley D, Cruz-Monserrate Z, Forsmark CE, et al. Type 3c (pancreatogenic) diabetes mellitus secondary to chronic pancreatitis and pancreatic cancer. Lancet Gastroenterol Hepatol. 2016;1(3):226-37.

[70] Rickels MR, Bellin M, Toledo FG, Robertson RP, Andersen DK, Chari ST, et al. Detection, evaluation and treatment of diabetes mellitus in chronic pancreatitis: recommendations from PancreasFest 2012. Pancreatology. 2013;13(4):336-42.

[71] Sheth SG, Conwell DL, Whitcomb DC, Alsante M, Anderson MA, Barkin J, et al. Academic Pancreas Centers of Excellence: Guidance from a multidisciplinary chronic pancreatitis working group at PancreasFest. Pancreatology. 2017;17(3):419-30.

[72] Bellin MD, Whitcomb DC, Abberbock J, Sherman S, Sandhu BS, Gardner TB, et al. Patient and Disease Characteristics Associated With the Presence of Diabetes Mellitus in Adults With Chronic Pancreatitis in the United States. Am J Gastroenterol. 2017;112(9):1457-65.

[73] Kumar K, Sharma R, Manrai M, Sood AK. Visceral Adipose Tissue as a Risk Factor for Diabetes Mellitus in Patients with Chronic Pancreatitis: A Cross-sectional, Observational Study. Diabetes Ther. 2017;8(5):1057-64.

[74] Wang W, Guo Y, Liao Z, Zou DW, Jin ZD, Zou DJ, et al. Occurrence of and risk factors for diabetes mellitus in Chinese patients with chronic

pancreatitis. Pancreas. 2011;40(2): 206-12.

[75] Mullady DK, Yadav D, Amann ST, O'Connell MR, Barmada MM, Elta GH, et al. Type of pain, pain-associated complications, quality of life, disability and resource utilisation in chronic pancreatitis: a prospective cohort study. Gut. 2011;60(1):77-84.

[76] Drewes AM, Olesen AE, Farmer AD, Szigethy E, Rebours V, Olesen SS. Gastrointestinal pain. Nat Rev Dis Primers. 2020;6(1):1.

[77] Anderson MA, Akshintala V, Albers KM, Amann ST, Belfer I, Brand R, et al. Mechanism, assessment and management of pain in chronic pancreatitis: Recommendations of a multidisciplinary study group. Pancreatology. 2016;16(1):83-94.

[78] Jadad AR, Browman GP. The WHO analgesic ladder for cancer pain management. Stepping up the quality of its evaluation. Jama. 1995;274(23): 1870-3.

[79] Juel J, Olesen SS, Olesen AE, Poulsen JL, Dahan A, Wilder-Smith O, et al. Study protocol for a randomised, double-blinded, placebo-controlled, clinical trial of S-ketamine for pain treatment in patients with chronic pancreatitis (RESET trial). BMJ Open. 2015;5(3):e007087.

[80] Olesen SS, Bouwense SA, Wilder-Smith OH, van Goor H, Drewes AM. Pregabalin reduces pain in patients with chronic pancreatitis in a randomized, controlled trial. Gastroenterology. 2011;141(2):536-43.

[81] Bhardwaj P, Garg PK, Maulik SK, Saraya A, Tandon RK, Acharya SK. A randomized controlled trial of antioxidant supplementation for pain relief in patients with chronic pancreatitis. Gastroenterology. 2009;136(1):149-59.e2.

[82] Rustagi T, Njei B. Antioxidant therapy for pain reduction in patients with chronic pancreatitis: a systematic review and meta-analysis. Pancreas. 2015;44(5):812-8.

[83] Siriwardena AK, Mason JM, Sheen AJ, Makin AJ, Shah NS. Antioxidant therapy does not reduce pain in patients with chronic pancreatitis: the ANTICIPATE study. Gastroenterology. 2012;143(3): 655-63.e1.

[84] Yaghoobi M, McNabb-Baltar J, Bijarchi R, Cotton PB. Pancreatic Enzyme Supplements Are Not Effective for Relieving Abdominal Pain in Patients with Chronic Pancreatitis: Meta-Analysis and Systematic Review of Randomized Controlled Trials. Can J Gastroenterol Hepatol. 2016;2016:8541839.

[85] Hoffmeister A, Mayerle J, Beglinger C, Büchler MW, Bufler P, Dathe K, et al. English language version of the S3-consensus guidelines on chronic pancreatitis: Definition, aetiology, diagnostic examinations, medical, endoscopic and surgical management of chronic pancreatitis. Z Gastroenterol. 2015;53(12):1447-95.

[86] Hookey LC, RioTinto R, Delhaye M, Baize M, Le Moine O, Devière J. Risk factors for pancreatitis after pancreatic sphincterotomy: a review of 572 cases. Endoscopy. 2006;38(7):670-6.

[87] Okolo PI, 3rd, Pasricha PJ, Kalloo AN. What are the long-term results of endoscopic pancreatic sphincterotomy? Gastrointest Endosc. 2000;52(1):15-9.

[88] Seza K, Yamaguchi T, Ishihara T, Tadenema H, Tawada K, Saisho H, et al. A long-term controlled trial of endoscopic pancreatic stenting for treatment of main pancreatic duct stricture in chronic pancreatitis.

Hepatogastroenterology. 2011;58(112):2128-31.

[89] Tringali A, Vadalà di Prampero SF, Landi R, Bove V, Familiari P, Hamanaka J, et al. Fully covered self-expandable metal stents to dilate persistent pancreatic strictures in chronic pancreatitis: long-term follow-up from a prospective study. Gastrointest Endosc. 2018;88(6):939-46.

[90] Cahen DL, van der Merwe SW, Laleman W, Poley JW, Bruno MJ. A biodegradable non-covered self-expandable stent to treat pancreatic duct strictures in chronic pancreatitis: a proof of principle. Gastrointest Endosc. 2018;87(2):486-91.

[91] Ahmed Ali U, Issa Y, Bruno MJ, van Goor H, van Santvoort H, Busch OR, et al. Early surgery versus optimal current step-up practice for chronic pancreatitis (ESCAPE): design and rationale of a randomized trial. BMC Gastroenterol. 2013;13:49.

[92] Drewes AM, Kempeneers MA, Andersen DK, Arendt-Nielsen L, Besselink MG, Boermeester MA, et al. Controversies on the endoscopic and surgical management of pain in patients with chronic pancreatitis: pros and cons! Gut. 2019;68(8):1343-51.

[93] Sarles H, Camarena J, Gomez-Santana C. Radiolucent and calcified pancreatic lithiasis: two different diseases. Role of alcohol and heredity. Scand J Gastroenterol. 1992;27(1):71-6.

[94] Widdison AL, Alvarez C, Karanjia ND, Reber HA. Experimental evidence of beneficial effects of ductal decompression in chronic pancreatitis. Endoscopy. 1991;23(3):151-4.

[95] Cahen DL, Gouma DJ, Laramée P, Nio Y, Rauws EA, Boermeester MA, et al. Long-term outcomes of endoscopic vs surgical drainage of the pancreatic duct in patients with chronic pancreatitis. Gastroenterology. 2011;141(5):1690-5.

[96] Ceyhan GO, Bergmann F, Kadihasanoglu M, Altintas B, Demir IE, Hinz U, et al. Pancreatic neuropathy and neuropathic pain--a comprehensive pathomorphological study of 546 cases. Gastroenterology. 2009;136(1):177-86.e1.

[97] Farnbacher MJ, Schoen C, Rabenstein T, Benninger J, Hahn EG, Schneider HT. Pancreatic duct stones in chronic pancreatitis: criteria for treatment intensity and success. Gastrointest Endosc. 2002;56(4):501-6.

[98] Dumonceau JM, Devière J, Le Moine O, Delhaye M, Vandermeeren A, Baize M, et al. Endoscopic pancreatic drainage in chronic pancreatitis associated with ductal stones: long-term results. Gastrointest Endosc. 1996;43(6):547-55.

[99] Ang TL. Chronic pancreatitis with pancreatic duct stricture and calculi treated by fully covered self-expandable metal stent placement and intraductal pancreatoscopy-guided laser lithotripsy. Endoscopy. 2017;49(6):E145-e6.

[100] Barthet M, Bugallo M, Moreira LS, Bastid C, Sastre B, Sahel J. Management of cysts and pseudocysts complicating chronic pancreatitis. A retrospective study of 143 patients. Gastroenterol Clin Biol. 1993;17(4):270-6.

[101] Andrén-Sandberg A, Dervenis C. Surgical treatment of pancreatic pseudocysts in the 2000's--laparoscopic approach. Acta Chir Iugosl. 2003;50(4):21-6.

[102] Ammann RW, Akovbiantz A, Largiader F, Schueler G. Course and outcome of chronic pancreatitis. Longitudinal study of a mixed medical-surgical series of 245 patients.

Gastroenterology. 1984;86(5 Pt 1): 820-8.

[103] Lerch MM, Stier A, Wahnschaffe U, Mayerle J. Pancreatic pseudocysts: observation, endoscopic drainage, or resection? Dtsch Arztebl Int. 2009;106(38):614-21.

[104] Barthet M, Lamblin G, Gasmi M, Vitton V, Desjeux A, Grimaud JC. Clinical usefulness of a treatment algorithm for pancreatic pseudocysts. Gastrointest Endosc. 2008;67(2):245-52.

[105] Panamonta N, Ngamruengphong S, Kijsirichareanchai K, Nugent K, Rakvit A. Endoscopic ultrasound-guided versus conventional transmural techniques have comparable treatment outcomes in draining pancreatic pseudocysts. Eur J Gastroenterol Hepatol. 2012;24(12):1355-62.

[106] Sriram PV, Kaffes AJ, Rao GV, Reddy DN. Endoscopic ultrasound-guided drainage of pancreatic pseudocysts complicated by portal hypertension or by intervening vessels. Endoscopy. 2005;37(3):231-5.

[107] Delhaye M, Matos C, Devière J. Endoscopic technique for the management of pancreatitis and its complications. Best Pract Res Clin Gastroenterol. 2004;18(1):155-81.

[108] Abdallah AA, Krige JE, Bornman PC. Biliary tract obstruction in chronic pancreatitis. HPB (Oxford). 2007;9(6):421-8.

[109] Barrioz T, Ingrand P, Besson I, de Ledinghen V, Silvain C, Beauchant M. Randomised trial of prevention of biliary stent occlusion by ursodeoxycholic acid plus norfloxacin. Lancet. 1994;344(8922):581-2.

[110] Ghosh S, Palmer KR. Prevention of biliary stent occlusion using cyclical antibiotics and ursodeoxycholic acid. Gut. 1994;35(12):1757-9.

[111] Catalano MF, Linder JD, George S, Alcocer E, Geenen JE. Treatment of symptomatic distal common bile duct stenosis secondary to chronic pancreatitis: comparison of single vs. multiple simultaneous stents. Gastrointest Endosc. 2004;60(6): 945-52.

[112] Singh VK, Yadav D, Garg PK. Diagnosis and Management of Chronic Pancreatitis: A Review. Jama. 2019;322(24):2422-34.

[113] Cahen DL, Gouma DJ, Nio Y, Rauws EA, Boermeester MA, Busch OR, et al. Endoscopic versus surgical drainage of the pancreatic duct in chronic pancreatitis. N Engl J Med. 2007;356(7):676-84.

[114] Olesen SS, Krauss T, Demir IE, Wilder-Smith OH, Ceyhan GO, Pasricha PJ, et al. Towards a neurobiological understanding of pain in chronic pancreatitis: mechanisms and implications for treatment. Pain Rep. 2017;2(6):e625.

[115] Tringali A, Bove V, Vadalà di Prampero SF, Boškoski I, Familiari P, Perri V, et al. Long-term follow-up after multiple plastic stenting for refractory pancreatic duct strictures in chronic pancreatitis. Endoscopy. 2019;51(10): 930-5.

[116] Laramée P, Wonderling D, Cahen DL, Dijkgraaf MG, Gouma DJ, Bruno MJ, et al. Trial-based cost-effectiveness analysis comparing surgical and endoscopic drainage in patients with obstructive chronic pancreatitis. BMJ Open. 2013;3(9):e003676.

[117] Kwon RS, Young BE, Marsteller WF, Lawrence C, Wu BU, Lee LS, et al. Narcotic Independence After Pancreatic Duct Stenting Predicts Narcotic Independence After Lateral Pancreaticojejunostomy for Chronic Pancreatitis. Pancreas. 2016;45(8): 1126-30.

[118] Olesen SS, Krarup H, Poulsen JL, Christensen JH, Sheel ARG, Sutton R, et al. Pancreas-specific plasma amylase for assessment and diagnosis of chronic pancreatitis: New insights on an old topic. United European Gastroenterol J. 2019;7(7):955-64.

[119] Beger HG, Schlosser W, Friess HM, Büchler MW. Duodenum-preserving head resection in chronic pancreatitis changes the natural course of the disease: a single-center 26-year experience. Ann Surg. 1999;230(4): 512-9; discussion 9-23.

[120] Plagemann S, Welte M, Izbicki JR, Bachmann K. Surgical Treatment for Chronic Pancreatitis: Past, Present, and Future. Gastroenterol Res Pract. 2017;2017:8418372.

[121] JC C. Chronic Pancreatitis — Update on Pathophysiology and Therapeutic Approaches. 2020.

[122] Bellin MD, Freeman ML, Gelrud A, Slivka A, Clavel A, Humar A, et al. Total pancreatectomy and islet autotransplantation in chronic pancreatitis: recommendations from PancreasFest. Pancreatology. 2014;14(1):27-35.

[123] Bellin MD, Forlenza GP, Majumder K, Berger M, Freeman ML, Beilman GJ, et al. Total Pancreatectomy With Islet Autotransplantation Resolves Pain in Young Children With Severe Chronic Pancreatitis. J Pediatr Gastroenterol Nutr. 2017;64(3):440-5.

[124] Chinnakotla S, Beilman GJ, Dunn TB, Bellin MD, Freeman ML, Radosevich DM, et al. Factors Predicting Outcomes After a Total Pancreatectomy and Islet Autotransplantation Lessons Learned From Over 500 Cases. Ann Surg. 2015;262(4):610-22.

[125] Kirkegård J, Mortensen FV, Cronin-Fenton D. Chronic Pancreatitis and Pancreatic Cancer Risk: A Systematic Review and Meta-analysis. Am J Gastroenterol. 2017;112(9): 1366-72.

[126] Domínguez-Muñoz JE, P DH, Lerch MM, Löhr MJ. Potential for Screening for Pancreatic Exocrine Insufficiency Using the Fecal Elastase-1 Test. Dig Dis Sci. 2017; 62(5):1119-30.

[127] Bekkali NL, Murray S, Johnson GJ, Bandula S, Amin Z, Chapman MH, et al. Pancreatoscopy-Directed Electrohydraulic Lithotripsy for Pancreatic Ductal Stones in Painful Chronic Pancreatitis Using SpyGlass. Pancreas. 2017;46(4):528-30.

[128] Domínguez-Muñoz JE. Pancreatic exocrine insufficiency: diagnosis and treatment. J Gastroenterol Hepatol. 2011;26 Suppl 2:12-6.

[129] Andersen DK, Korc M, Petersen GM, Eibl G, Li D, Rickels MR, et al. Diabetes, Pancreatogenic Diabetes, and Pancreatic Cancer. Diabetes. 2017;66(5):1103-10.

[130] Duggan SN, Purcell C, Kilbane M, O'Keane M, McKenna M, Gaffney P, et al. An association between abnormal bone turnover, systemic inflammation, and osteoporosis in patients with chronic pancreatitis: a case-matched study. Am J Gastroenterol. 2015;110(2): 336-45.

[131] Sikkens EC, Cahen DL, Koch AD, Braat H, Poley JW, Kuipers EJ, et al. The prevalence of fat-soluble vitamin deficiencies and a decreased bone mass in patients with chronic pancreatitis. Pancreatology. 2013;13(3):238-42.

[132] Bang UC, Benfield T, Bendtsen F, Hyldstrup L, Beck Jensen JE. The risk of fractures among patients with cirrhosis or chronic pancreatitis. Clin Gastroenterol Hepatol. 2014;12(2): 320-6.

[133] Hao L, Zeng XP, Xin L, Wang D, Pan J, Bi YW, et al. Incidence of and risk factors for pancreatic cancer in chronic pancreatitis: A cohort of 1656 patients. Dig Liver Dis. 2017;49(11):1249-56.

[134] Algül H, Treiber M, Lesina M, Schmid RM. Mechanisms of disease: chronic inflammation and cancer in the pancreas--a potential role for pancreatic stellate cells? Nat Clin Pract Gastroenterol Hepatol. 2007;4(8): 454-62.

[135] Tamura K, Yu J, Hata T, Suenaga M, Shindo K, Abe T, et al. Mutations in the pancreatic secretory enzymes CPA1 and CPB1 are associated with pancreatic cancer. Proc Natl Acad Sci U S A. 2018;115(18):4767-72.

[136] Goggins M, Overbeek KA, Brand R, Syngal S, Del Chiaro M, Bartsch DK, et al. Management of patients with increased risk for familial pancreatic cancer: updated recommendations from the International Cancer of the Pancreas Screening (CAPS) Consortium. Gut. 2020;69(1):7-17.

[137] Whitcomb DC, Shelton CA, Brand RE. Genetics and Genetic Testing in Pancreatic Cancer. Gastroenterology. 2015;149(5):1252-64.e4.

[138] Hao W, Komar HM, Hart PA, Conwell DL, Lesinski GB, Friedman A. Mathematical model of chronic pancreatitis. Proc Natl Acad Sci U S A. 2017;114(19):5011-6.

[139] Chari ST, Mohan V, Pitchumoni CS, Viswanathan M, Madanagopalan N, Lowenfels AB. Risk of pancreatic carcinoma in tropical calcifying pancreatitis: an epidemiologic study. Pancreas. 1994;9(1):62-6.